Table of Contents

D0904715

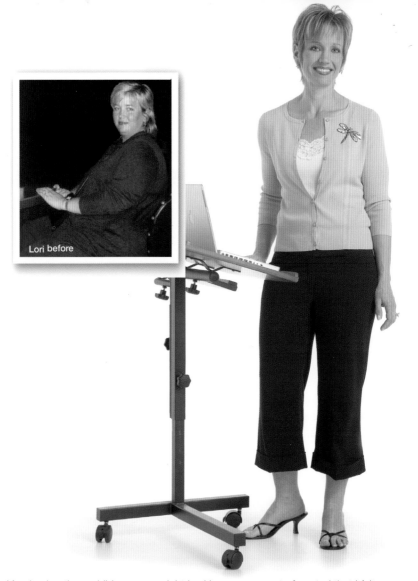

Lori before

After having three children, my weight had become so out of control that I felt completely overwhelmed. I tried several diets until my weight crept to an all time high. I decided to log onto the Jenny Craig website and learn more about the program. I was so motivated by the success stories, that I called the local Jenny Craig Centre and never looked back. It was inspiring to know that my consultant believed in me and would be with me every step of the way. Plus, I never felt deprived. The food was tasty and I was still able to eat and cook with my family! Jenny Craig was a plan I could stick to. And now look at me, I am 100 pounds lighter!

Lori S.
lost a total of 100* pounds with Jenny Craig
*Results not typical.

*Welcome to Jenny **Your**Style*®

Congratulations on making the commitment to achieve your healthy weight goal. You're about to embark on a journey of self-discovery where you'll learn about your current beliefs and behaviors regarding food and physical activity and explore new ones that will enable you to manage your weight for life. It's our goal to provide you with the basics of nutrition and physical activity, so you have the information, skills and strategies you need for successful weight loss and well-being.

This guide will help you through the first few weeks of your program with an introduction to the weight loss process and information on the three success factors: Food, Body and Mind. This guide also contains more information on how we will be using **Your**Style® Profile results to tailor your program.

To keep things simple in the first few weeks of your program, we've pared it down to the essentials. However, if you have additional questions, please feel free to ask your consultant or centre director. They're here to support you all the way.

What's Contributed to Your Weight Challenges?

As a client embarking on the weight loss journey, you bring along not only your weight loss history, but also your beliefs about that history. For instance, do you believe that:

- The cause of your weight challenges is biological – that your genetics have made you overweight?
- It's environmental – that there are too many food choices to resist and too few opportunities to be active at home or at work?
- Your hectic lifestyle or personal motivation gets in the way of healthy choices?
- It's confusion about the facts regarding what to eat and how to exercise for successful weight loss that keeps you from your goals?

Experts say that, the truth is, all these factors play a role in weight. Some factors, like genetics, can't be radically changed, but many others like the environment, lifestyle, motivation and knowledge are all under your control. Interestingly, research suggests that believing in your ability to control your weight can actually help you to succeed with your goal*. The fact that you are deciding to work on your weight says you do have some belief in your ability to manage it.

*Wamsteker EW, Geenen R, Iestra J, et al. Obesity-related beliefs predict weight loss after an 8-week low-calorie diet. J Am Diet Assoc. 1995;105:441-444.

What Motivates You?

Deciding to enroll in Jenny Craig was your first step on the journey to weight loss and well being. Celebrate the decision and ask yourself how your life will be different. What personal benefits – besides weight loss – are you looking for in the weeks to come?

What areas of your life are most important to you?

☐ Appearance   ☐ Family   ☐ Relationships   ☐ Activities
☐ Health   ☐ Career   ☐ Self-Image

Fuel Motivation with Visualization
Motivation is what fuels your desire to move along the path to meet your goals. It's simply the powerful feelings that propel you to make healthy changes.

Take a moment to visualize how you will feel when you reach your weight goal and realize the benefits that matter most to you.
Will you feel…?

☐ Energized   ☐ In Control   ☐ Other

☐ Proud   ☐ Empowered   ☐ _____

☐ Self-Confident   ☐ At Peace   ☐ _____

Every day, take a moment to paint that mental picture of your personal benefits and the deeply powerful feelings you associate with them.
Each week, expand your vision a little more, to include seeing yourself in a variety of situations – dining out, shopping, working, socializing, being active, taking advantage of new opportunities, etc. As you move along the path to your goal, the growing vision of your benefits and feelings will re-affirm your healthy choices and fuel your motivation to maintain your healthy changes.

You've Made the Right Choice

A Comprehensive Solution
By choosing Jenny Craig, you've chosen an approach to weight loss that is based on sound, scientific research. Designed by our staff of registered dietitians in consultation with an expert Medical Advisory Board, the Jenny Craig **Your**Style® Program takes a comprehensive approach to weight management that includes the three success factors:

Food: A Healthy Relationship with Food
Body: An Active Lifestyle
Mind: A Balanced Approach to Living

A Healthy Solution
And, when you make the change to a healthy lifestyle, the benefits extend beyond weight loss. By losing as little as 5-10% of your weight, as the individuals in the study on the next page did, you can reduce your risk for heart disease, hypertension, diabetes and certain cancers.

Each of the success factors plays a role in disease prevention:

Food
A menu rich in fruits, vegetables, whole grains and reduced fat dairy products may reduce your risk for heart disease, hypertension and cancer.

Body
Consistent physical activity may lower your risk for heart disease, diabetes and cancer.

Mind
Positive coping skills and stress management skills may enhance your immunity, as well as reduce your blood pressure, anxiety and heart disease risk.

A Record of Success
For over 20 years, Jenny Craig has been recognized as a leading provider of successful, healthy weight loss results. The Cooper Institute conducted an analysis of 60,164 men and women who enrolled in at least a one-year Program between May 2001 and May 2002.*

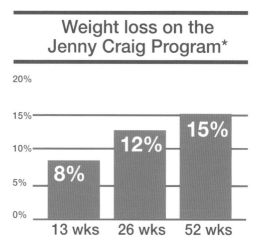

Weight loss on the Jenny Craig Program*

	13 wks	26 wks	52 wks
	8%	12%	15%

*Based on observational data of clients who enrolled in at least a one-year program and attended at least 85% of their weekly consultations. Of those clients who enrolled in the one-year program, 42% remained at 13 weeks, 22% at 26 weeks and 6.6% at 52 weeks. Finley CE, Barlow CE, Greenway FL, et al. Retention rates and weight loss in a commercial weight loss program. *Int J Obes* (Lon). 2007;31:292-298.

Jenny Craig's YourStyle®: A total approach to healthy weight loss that works!

Support Makes the Difference

Think of us as partners in a lifestyle change. We'll walk with you on your journey to weight loss. In your weekly consultations, we'll celebrate your "Wins," work through your challenges, and build on your success.

Tell a Friend, and You Win

Studies show that having the support of others can help you stay on the weight loss course. Researchers compared people who joined a weight loss program with family members or friends to those who joined alone. Ninety-seven percent of those with support completed the program, while only 76% of those who joined solo followed through*. Having support can make a difference! Who do you know who could benefit from losing weight? Ask your consultant about our Guest Promotions.

We're Here for You

At Jenny Craig, we are here to provide you with the highest quality service. If you need to make a switch—either in your appointment or with your consultant—just give us 24-hours' notice. That's what one-on-one support is all about! Speaking of 24 hours, you can also call our complimentary customer care line at 1-800-JennyCare to answer your questions or discuss your concerns 24 hours a day, seven days a week. If you're unable to reach your consultant during regular business hours or are phoning when your centre is closed, just call JennyCare for a quick, friendly answer to your question.

You're Never Alone

Check out our supportive online community and connect with others who share your commitment. Message Boards and Chat Rooms at jennycraig.com are a wonderful way to meet new friends and get encouragement when you need it most. And "What's Your Motivation?" lets you share tips to stay on track. As a Jenny Craig client, you have free access to all of the Online Tools, including the Menu Planner, Recipes, Progress Tracker, Activity Planner, Journal, and Affirmations. You can also choose to receive a weekly newsletter and tips via email. Visit jennycraig.com today!

---

*Wing RR, Jeffery RW. Benefits of recruiting participants with friends and increasing social support for weight loss and maintenance. *J Consult Clin Psychol*. 1999;67:132-138.

Understanding the Weight Loss Process

Weight loss is a process; it happens in phases. Understanding these phases will help you know what to expect, how to set goals and when to make adjustments in your weekly plan. Here's an overview of the process, which all starts with the concept of balance.

Weight Loss is a Matter of Balance

Losing weight may seem complicated, but it really comes down to this: take in fewer calories than your body burns every day. Following your Jenny Craig Menu as you increase your physical activity can tip the scales in your favor.

The Energy Balance Equation

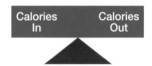

| Jenny Craig Menu | Calories In | Calories Out | Resting Metabolism and Physical Activity |

Calories In: Food

Calories come from carbohydrate, fat, protein or alcohol. Although water, vitamins and minerals are essential nutrients, they do not contain any calories. To simplify calorie control, you have the benefit of pre-portioned Jenny's Cuisine as part of a lowfat, calorie-reduced menu.

Calories Out: Body

Your body is always burning calories because calories are used to create the energy that your body needs to function. Everything you do requires calories—breathing, moving, thinking, speaking and even digesting food.

The amount of energy your body burns when you are at rest is called your resting metabolism. Resting metabolism is determined by your gender, height, weight, age and body composition. It is usually higher in men, due to a higher percentage of muscle, which naturally burns more calories. Resting metabolism may decrease with age, due to muscle loss from decreased activity. It may also decrease as you lose weight, because a smaller body requires fewer calories. Your body also burns calories through physical activity. In combination with eating fewer calories, calories burned from activity can make a big difference in both weight loss and maintenance.

What About Your Calorie Output and Menu Level?

When you enrolled in Jenny Craig, your gender, height, weight and age were entered into a computer that calculates your resting metabolism. This number was multiplied by an activity factor to determine your total calorie output. That number was used to calculate your Jenny Craig weight loss menu.

As a reference, eating an extra 3500 calories results in a one pound weight gain. So, if you reduce your calorie intake by 500 every day, in a week, you'd typically lose one pound. Your menu level has been calculated to result in approximately one to two pounds of weekly weight loss.

Determining a Healthy Weight Range

To help you select your desired weight goal, we've identified a healthy weight range based on a body mass index (BMI) of 19-24. BMI is both an indicator of weight and health. BMI is affected by body composition. If you are a man, large-boned or very muscular, your desired weight may be at the higher end of your healthy weight range. Reducing your weight closer to this range reduces your risk for conditions such as heart disease, diabetes and cancer.

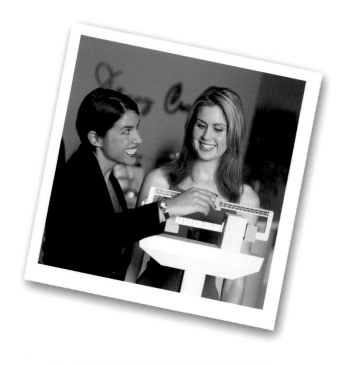

Food

Dispelling the Myths

With so many popular diets and so much dieting information out there today, it can be difficult to separate fact from fiction. Let's take a look at some commonly held food myths, and the facts to dispel them...

Myth: Certain foods can help burn fat.
Fact: There are no foods with magic fat-burning ingredients. Some foods with caffeine temporarily speed up your metabolism, but probably not enough to lead to weight loss.

Myth: Cutting out starches is the best way to lose weight.
Fact: The best way to lose weight is to follow a balanced plan that you can stick with for the long-term, and, of course, to burn more calories than you eat. (Remember the energy balance equation). Eliminating food groups reduces your intake of nutrients that are important for your health, and restrictive diets are difficult to follow over the long-term. So it's important to design a balanced menu to match your personal taste and lifestyle. While some people prefer to include their favorite starches/desserts, others are more satisfied by protein-rich foods. That is why Jenny Craig offers a customized carbohydrate approach. You have the option of selecting higher protein menu items, noted with a ⬆ in your Personalized Menu Planner. You can select foods you prefer, knowing that you are following a healthy plan that will work for you long-term.

Myth: I shouldn't eat any fat.
Fact: Fat serves many important functions, such as storing energy, transporting certain vitamins and providing flavor and texture to foods. When it comes to weight loss, calories are the bottom line. Reduced-fat foods often have reduced calories compared to their full-fat counterparts. But, be sure to check the label, as some reduced-fat or fat-free foods have added sugar to maintain their flavor, which increases the calories. When it comes to health, moderate fat intake (20-35% of your calories) is recommended, mostly from unsaturated sources. (See page 14 for more information).

Myth: Eating after 8:00 p.m. leads to weight gain.
Fact: Your body burns food the same way no matter what time it is. What matters is: what you eat, how much you eat and how active you are. No matter when you eat, excess calories will be stored as fat. If you are eating high calorie/high fat foods while watching late night television, you may gain weight because of your food choices, not due to the time of day. Also, snacking while doing other things like watching television can easily lead to overeating because distractions may cause you to lose track of how much you are eating.

Myth: Skipping meals will help me lose weight.
Fact: If you skip meals, you will probably be more likely to snack or eat more at your next meal, consuming more calories than you would if you had not skipped a meal.

Myth: I can only lose weight if I eat less than 1000 calories per day.
Fact: Consuming too few calories can send your body into "starvation mode." Your metabolism slows down, putting your body into a state of survival in which it conserves more of the calories you eat, making it more difficult for you to lose weight.

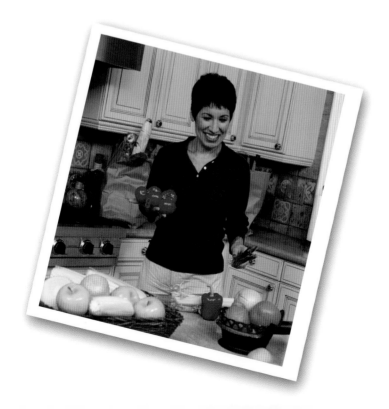

The Value of Your Menu

The 2005 Dietary Guidelines for Americans say a healthy diet:
- Emphasizes fruits, vegetables, whole grains and reduced fat milk products.
- Includes lean meats, poultry, fish, beans, eggs, and nuts.
- Promotes heart healthy fats and limits saturated fats, trans fats, cholesterol, salt (sodium) and added sugars.

These diet guidelines are reflected in your Jenny Craig Menus, which are designed by Jenny Craig's registered dietitians.

The Benefits of Portion Control

Your menu features a variety of prepared entrées and snacks which are convenient models for nutritional balance, variety and portion control.

Did you know...?
- Between 1977 and 1996, average food portions increased dramatically, especially for foods eaten at fast-food restaurants and at home.[1]

- When we're served larger portions, we tend to eat more. In one study, people consumed 30% more food when offered a larger portion, even though they were just as satisfied with a smaller portion.[2]

- Our ability to "eyeball" portion size is not very good, so having a pre-portioned "unit" of food provides a visual model and controls calories.

- Research has shown that pre-packaged meals can be more effective in helping people lose weight and reduce heart disease risk compared to people preparing their own meals on a conventional weight loss plan.[3]

So, not only does Jenny's Cuisine give you a convenient model of portion size, it may also be a tool to help you feel satisfied in a healthy way!

[1] Nielsen SJ, Popkin BM. Patterns and trends in food portion sizes, 1977-1998. *JAMA*. 2003;289:450-453.

[2] Rolls BJ, Morris EL, Roe LS. Portion size of food affects energy intake in normal-weight and overweight men and women. *Am J Clin Nutr*. 2002;76:1207-1213.

[3] Hannum SM, Carson L, Evans EM, et al. Use of portion-controlled entrees enhances weight loss in women. *Obesity Res*. 2004;12:538-546.

Setting Up Your Menu

- Check off the foods as you eat to easily track your intake, making note of any foods missed or extra foods eaten.
- Learn about nutritional balance, variety and moderation in portion sizes with Jenny's Cuisine.
- Refer to Jenny's Grocery List on page 70 to tailor your menu to your lifestyle and taste.
- Use the Grocery List as a guide to serving size for a variety of different foods.
- Make shopping easy with the "My Own Foods" list on the back of your Menu. It can be as simple as:

2 sacks of fruit
2 bags of pre-washed/frozen vegetables
2 bags of salad greens
1 gallon of nonfat milk
1 jar peanut butter

- Stay satisfied and add variety to your week with Free Foods in the "Personalize Your Menu" section of your menu.
- Dining out or cooking at home? Follow the food groups in the "Meal on My Own" section to keep your calories within a consistent range.
- Complement your Menu with your Jenny Craig supplements/bar every day.

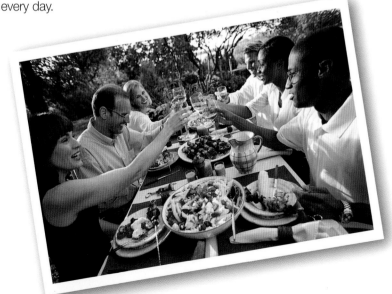

Grocery Foods

At Jenny Craig, you're learning about portion control, balance and variety in food choices. Your Jenny Craig Menu features a healthy balance between Jenny's Cuisine and your own grocery foods. Here is an overview to enable you to make the best choices within each group.

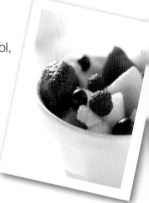

Vegetables and Fruit
- Each day of your menu includes at least three vegetable and two fruit servings.
- Fruits and vegetables are important sources of fiber, vitamins, minerals and phytonutrients.
- Eat "across the rainbow" for health benefits—enjoy a variety of colors (orange, red, dark green, etc.) in order to get a variety of   nutrients.
- Mix up your salad greens, alternating romaine, spinach, watercress, etc. with lighter-leafed lettuce choices.
- To maintain healthy blood pressure, choose potassium-rich vegetables such as beet greens, tomatoes and spinach and potassium-rich fruits, such as bananas, cantaloupe, honeydew, dried peaches/apricots and oranges.
- Non-starchy vegetables and certain fruits, which are low in calories are "free" – eat all you like! (See page 15 for more information on Free Foods).
- Non-starchy vegetables include all vegetables except: corn, peas, potatoes, winter squash and yams, which belong to the starch group.
- A Garden Salad is a free food and can be made with any of your favorite assorted, chopped vegetables on a bed of shredded lettuce, mixed greens and/or spinach.

Meats
- Meats and meat substitutes are important sources of protein. The "Meat" group also contains meatless sources of protein, such as beans, cheese and tofu.
- Higher fat meats should be consumed in moderation because they are high in saturated fat and cholesterol—which may contribute to heart disease.
- Fish, such as tuna, salmon and mackerel, can be a good source of omega-three fatty acids, which may protect against heart disease, arthritis and Alzheimer's disease.

Milk
- Every day, your Jenny Craig Menu has an equivalent of 2 to 4 cups of nonfat milk/yogurt, depending on your calorie level.
- Milk and yogurt are good sources of calcium, which helps protect your bones and prevent osteoporosis.
- Dairy products have also been shown to support weight loss in clinical studies[1].
- You can use an Anytime Bar* to replace one of your milk servings and your supplements.
- If you're lactose intolerant, try one of these ideas.
    - Divide one cup milk into two, half cup servings.
    - Buy lactose reduced, nonfat milk.
    - You can also exchange for one cup nonfat milk:
        - 1 Anytime Bar*
        - 1 cup nonfat yogurt or butter/soy milk   • 2 egg whites**
        - 1 oz lowfat cheese or lean meat**   • 1/4 cup light tofu**

* Limit to 1 Bar per day (U.S. only).
** To meet your calcium needs, be sure to take your Jenny Craig Supplements.

[1] Zemel MB, Thompson W, Milstead A, et al. Calcium and dairy acceleration of weight and fat loss during energy restriction in obese adults. *Obesity Res*. 2004;12:582-590.

Starches
- Starches, including bread, cereal, corn, pasta, potato, rice and other grains, provide fuel for all your cells.
- High fiber foods can help you feel more satisfied without adding extra calories.
- Whole grain starches provide fiber and a variety of other nutrients which can protect against heart disease, diabetes and certain cancers and digestive disorders.
- Examples of whole grains include brown rice, buckwheat, bulgur, oatmeal, wild rice, whole rye, whole-grain barley, and whole wheat berries, bread, crackers, pasta and tortillas.
- Look for grain products that:
    - List whole/sprouted/malted/cracked wheat or other whole grain as the first ingredient.
    - Contain at least 2 grams of fiber per serving.
- To maintain healthy blood pressure, choose potassium-rich starchy vegetables like sweet potatoes, white beans, soybeans, winter squash, lentils, kidney beans and split peas.

Fat

- For weight loss, it is a good idea to moderate your intake of all types of fat, because a gram of fat contains more than twice the calories of a gram of protein or carbohydrate.
- To reduce your heart risk, choose mostly unsaturated fats over saturated fats and limit intake of trans fats and cholesterol (see charts).
- Jenny's Cuisine has been specially formulated to be low in saturated fat, cholesterol and trans fat.

Fats that Raise Cholesterol and Risk of Heart Disease	Significant Sources	Examples
Dietary Cholesterol	Foods from animals	Higher fat meats and higher fat milks
Saturated Fats	Foods from animals	Higher fat meats and higher fat milks
	Palm, palm kernel and coconut oils and cocoa butter	Some higher fat starches, such as cookies, crackers, chips and candy
Trans Fats	Partially hydrogenated vegetable oils	Margarine and shortening, cookies, crackers, cakes and commercial fried foods

Adapted from the American Heart Association. www.americanheart.org

[1] Zemel MB, Thompson W, Milstead A, et al. Calcium and dairy acceleration of weight and fat loss during energy restriction in obese adults. *Obesity Res*. 2004;12:582-590.

Fats that Lower Cholesterol	Sources	Examples
Polyunsaturated Fats	Certain plant oils, nuts and seeds	Safflower, pumpkin, soy, corn and sunflower
Monounsaturated Fats	Certain plant oils, nuts and seeds	Olive, canola, peanut, sesame, almond, cashew, pecan and avocados

Adapted from the American Heart Association. www.americanheart.org

- For the added fats on your menu, choose fats and oils:
    - With 2 grams or less saturated fat per tablespoon with 0 grams trans fat
    - As liquid/tub margarines
    - Derived from poly/monounsaturated sources
- Vary your choices with heart-healthy nuts/seeds, avocadoes or whole olives.

Free Foods

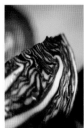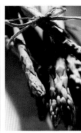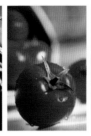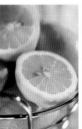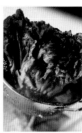

Free foods are a great way to add both flavor and satisfaction to your Menu. See your Grocery List or the back of your Menus for a variety of low or no calorie ideas.

Free Foods – Unlimited
You can enjoy unlimited amounts of non-starchy vegetables, such as tomatoes, cucumbers, onions and mushrooms – for variety and satisfaction. You can also enjoy calorie-free beverages, sugar substitutes, flavor enhancers such as herbs and spices, sugar-free gelatin dessert and sugar-free gum (see Jenny's Grocery List, page 74).

Free Foods – Limited
(Choose up to 3 servings per day)
While these foods are still low-calorie (each provides < 30 calories per serving), you'll want to limit them to keep your daily calories consistent.
• Strawberries, cantaloupe, watermelon and grapefruit (1/2 cup, each) are healthy examples of limited free foods.
• Sugar-free candy, whipped topping or syrup and some fat-free condiments also fall into this category (see Jenny's Grocery List, page 74).

Water and Other Beverages

Why Water?
Water carries nutrients to the cells and transports wastes to the kidneys and lungs for excretion. Water also cushions joints and tissues, aids digestion and assists in temperature regulation. Water is one of a weight manager's best tools—take a sip, quench your thirst and you'll often find it wasn't food, but fluid, that you needed. Did you know that water is a great energy enhancer? Thirst and dehydration can cause fatigue. So, drink up for an extra dose of vitality!

Water Tips on Tap
- Snap up the flavor with a slice of lemon or a squeeze of lime.
- At work, keep a full glass at your desk.
- Before you eat, drink a glass of water.
- Try club soda, sparkling, mineral or calorie-free flavored water.

Other Beverages

Coffee/Tea/Soft Drinks
If you are a heavy coffee or tea drinker, consider cutting back if it interferes with your milk or water intake. If you do decide to cut back on caffeine, do so gradually–cutting your intake in half each week, to avoid caffeine-withdrawal related symptoms.

Common Caffeine Counts

Beverage	Amount	Caffeine (mg)
Coffee	6 oz	104
Decaffeinated Coffee	6 oz	10
Brewed Tea	6 oz	35
Diet Cola	12 oz	50
Hot Chocolate	6 oz	5
Tall Coffee Drink*	12 oz	75
Grande Coffee Drink*	16 oz	150
Vente Coffee Drink (hot)	20 oz	150
Vente Coffee Drink (cold)	20 oz	70

(*Includes cappuccino, latte, Americano)

Alcohol
Alcohol provides calories with minimal nutrients, so consider reducing your intake during weight loss.
- If you choose to drink alcohol, consider limiting intake to two servings per week.
- Also, you can increase activity to offset the calories.
- If you choose to drink more, you can work with your consultant to balance your menu.
- If you have diabetes or other health conditions, consult your physician regarding your alcohol intake.

Calorie Count of Alcoholic Beverages

Beverage	Amount	Calories
Wine (red/rosé/white)	5 oz	110
Wine Spritzer (half wine/half soda)	5 oz	55
Beer	12 oz	150
Distilled Spirits	1 oz	100
Martini	2 oz	156

Your Jenny Craig Supplements

Experts say it's very difficult to get all the vitamins, minerals and other nutrients you need on a reduced calorie menu. To ensure that you receive the balanced nutrition you need during weight loss, it's essential that you complement your Jenny Craig Menu with your Jenny Craig Supplements.*

Anytime Vitamin Bar*

This delicious supplement was especially prepared to complement the Jenny Craig Menu, providing a spectrum of nutrients, including iron, calcium, folic acid and vitamin E, the quantities of which may be reduced on a calorie-restricted menu. This convenient bar can be enjoyed any time of the day as a replacement for one cup nonfat milk/yogurt on your Jenny Craig Menu.

MultiPlus*

This multivitamin/mineral supplement also provides the full range of vitamins and minerals necessary during weight loss. MultiPlus is designed to be taken with a glass of water in the morning and evening. If you're sensitive to supplements, try taking them with your two larger meals (lunch and dinner).

ProTect Plus*

This special antioxidant formula gives added protection against body cell damage due to sunlight, cigarette smoke, air pollution and even the normal oxidative process of aging. What's the "plus"? Extra phytonutrients, derived from natural vegetable extracts, provide additional nutrients for optimal health.

For Canadian Clients

Every day, your Jenny Craig Menu includes a delicious Jenny Craig Bar or Drink, which provides valuable vitamins and minerals, along with calories, protein, carbohydrate and fat. To ensure your complete nutritional balance, enjoy one every day!

*U.S. only

Your Typical Meal Pattern

Your typical meal pattern is a reflection of your lifestyle, habits and preferences. You may prefer small, frequent meals or snacks to keep you going, or you may find that frequent eating increases temptation, takes too much time/planning, or you would just rather have three more substantial meals. Not skipping meals is important because it may lead to overeating when you do eat; there is no magic number of meals and snacks to eat for weight loss.

The Value of Self-Monitoring

Over and over, research has shown that those who self-monitor are more successful with lifestyle change. In fact, in one famous study, those who kept a food log over the holidays actually lost weight, without even being on a diet. This evidence shows that the act of tracking, logging, keeping a diary, etc. can actually influence and change your choices.

Why? Because the moment you take to write down what you eat or how much activity you engage in is a decision point. You may choose to eat less, or choose not to eat at all. You may choose to maintain your current step goal or be so energized by the feelings you have afterward that you increase your goal by 2000 steps the next day.

Your Jenny Craig Menu has been especially designed to be a convenient self-monitoiring tool. In the next several weeks, you'll learn just how easy it is to track a variety of food/body/mind behaviors. Whichever ones you choose to track, know that the value it is not in catching yourself making "bad" choices. It's in building your awareness of *what* drives your choices as well as what positive choices you *are* making. Both are the foundation for developing a healthy, balanced lifestyle.

Common Questions

The following questions are commonly asked by new clients. If you have others, feel free to ask your consultant or centre director— they're there for you!

Q: Why are weekly consultations recommended?
A: Research has shown that frequent contact enhances weight loss and many clients credit weekly consultations for their success. Weekly weigh-ins also ensure a safe rate of weight loss and enable your consultant to offer strategies to help you meet your goals.

Q: Can I choose my own foods?
A: Yes, our Personalized Menu is designed to let you choose the foods you like. You started on the menu that your profile indicated may work best for your lifestyle, but you may switch between planned and personalized menus as desired.

Q: What if I don't care for one of the grocery foods on my menu?
A: Any food not listed in boldfaced type on your menu may easily be traded for another in the same food group. See the Jenny's Grocery List in the back of this guide or ask your consultant for suggestions.

Q: What if I don't want salad?
A: You can substitute sliced raw vegetables (great for dipping in Jenny's Dressing), stir-fry raw vegetables with a teaspoon of olive oil or find alternative recipes for a vegetable and a fat serving in the Jenny Craig cookbooks. Remember, it's okay to have extra non-starchy vegetables because they're free.

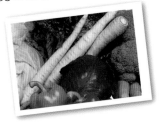

Q: Can I change consultants?
A: Yes, if you feel that another consultant may be better suited to meet your needs, just call the centre. We're here to help you succeed. Your consultant serves as coach, confidante and motivator, so it's important to be comfortable with your consultant.

Q: How do I handle dining out or special occasions?
A: Built into your menu is a "Meal on My Own" section that gives you a list of foods/portion sizes for breakfast, lunch and dinner options to keep your calories consistent with your Jenny Craig Menu.

Developing a Healthy Relationship with Food

Food means different things to different people; it nourishes the body, pleases the taste buds, and comforts the soul. Experiences throughout your life have been shaping your relationship with food – from your childhood mealtime rituals, to your school nutrition class, to your past dieting attempts – all of these things factor in to your food choices today. You also eat for a variety of reasons; it may be in response to internal cues, like physical hunger and emotions, or it may be in response to external cues like time, place, social activities and specific events. Your Eating Style reflects some of your individual experiences, eating cues and habits in order to identify the strategies that will work for you. Whether you are already a balanced eater, or you have a variety of eating styles, you will learn to eat enjoyably and healthfully throughout the program.

What's Your Eating Style?

Learn more about your personal eating styles by referring to the sections that correspond to YourStyle® Profile results...

Uninformed Eater – learning about healthy eating
• You have the best intentions, but maybe not the best information. See page 21.

Emotional Eater – eating in response to feelings
• In the moment, you may respond to your feelings instead of your physical hunger cues. See page 22.

Unconscious Eater – unaware of your eating
• You may miss meals, eat meals while doing other things, or eat something just because "it's there." See page 23.

Social Eater – influenced by others
• You may be tempted to eat by a variety of people, places and events. See page 24.

Balanced Eater – maintaining a healthy relationship with food
• You are able to make nutritious choices and balance them with the pleasure of eating. See page 25.

The Styles

Uninformed Eater

Goal: Learn about healthy food choices.

Focus on a Healthy, Non-Diet Approach

When it comes to healthy eating for weight loss, you have the best of intentions. You're up on the latest diets; in fact, you've tried a lot of them. You may be very interested in nutrition and motivated to eat healthfully. Or, you may have a set of "dieting" habits that you think support weight loss, but you're not getting any closer to your goal. These habits may include cutting out carbs, counting fat grams or eliminating your favorite foods. In fact, your efforts to restrict "bad" foods may backfire on you, as it's tough to follow restrictive plans for very long, and the "rebound" overeating that often occurs leaves you weighing more than before.

Mastering Uninformed Eating

The good news is, you don't have to do anything extreme to reach your goals. Experts say that successful weight loss is a matter of calorie control, and the key to calorie control is portion control. During your program, you'll be using the model of Jenny's Cuisine to learn about correct portion sizes as you eat a variety of foods.

Keeping Track

Use your Jenny Craig Menu and Jenny's Cuisine as a learning and self-monitoring tool. This week, notice the mix of foods that make up your meals – lean protein, fresh fruits and vegetables, lowfat dairy products and heart-healthy fats. Keep a tally of the food groups as you eat them. Also, notice the portion sizes of Jenny's Cuisine entrées and snacks. How do they compare to your old serving sizes and the serving sizes of your favorite restaurants? Self-monitoring your food intake for balance and moderation will be a key factor in your weight loss and weight maintenance success.

Emotional Eater

Goal: Learn to eat in response to your hunger cues.

Focus on Breaking the Cycle

One of the most difficult challenges many weight managers face is trying to
eat healthfully when experiencing strong emotions. Like many emotional
eaters, you may resort to food to calm, soothe, or even squelch your feelings.
In the moment, you may not respond to your physical hunger cues, or even
care as much about your healthy eating goal. Instead, you may feel driven by
the emotional need to feel comforted. If you do have a slip, you might feel
upset and guilty about it, and those negative feelings might lead to a binge or
giving up on your plan. In fact, one reason you may overeat in response to
emotions is that you're overly restrictive with what you eat. Establishing a
regular pattern of eating and avoiding depriving yourself of your favorite foods
can be helpful.

Mastering Emotional Eating

To break the cycle, it's important to understand the link between your
emotions, thoughts and actions. In the weeks ahead, you'll be learning to do
just that. For this week, if you feel yourself being swept away in a sea of
emotions and headed straight for food, re-gain control by mentally telling
yourself to "STOP!" and ask yourself what you really need.
Ask yourself ….
    Do I need…
            Food to nourish me?
            Physical activity to re-energize me?
            Rest to rejuvenate me?
            A talk to express my emotions?
            Relaxation to soothe my tension?
            A deep breath to restore my calm?
    If food isn't what you need, consider an alternative.

Keeping Track

In the "Why" section under "Extra Foods Eaten" on your menu, note what
feelings, if any, drive you to eat. Is it hunger, anger, stress, excitement,
boredom or fatigue that drives your choices? Are there healthy alternatives
you want to plan into your next week as a result? If you don't follow your plan
exactly, pay attention to your thoughts and feelings and use it as a learning
opportunity. Identifying the places, events and feelings that cue you to eat,
will help you create successful plans for nonfood ways to manage your
feelings in the future.

Unconscious Eater

Goal: Develop self-awareness.

Focus on Self-Awareness

In a busy, stressful world, it's easy to see how you might develop the habit of unconscious eating, where you're not truly aware of how much or even what you're eating over the course of the day. As an unconscious eater, you typically miss meals, eat meals while doing other things, or just graze your way throughout the day. You might even find yourself eating something just because "it's there," or because you grew up in a family where everyone just naturally "cleaned their plate." If so, know that you're not alone. The first step to a new relationship with food is self-awareness – understanding your current patterns, so that you can make healthy changes and actually enjoy the pleasure of eating more.

Mastering Unconscious Eating

Begin to notice your hunger and satisfaction signals; be aware of portion size and the mix of foods on your menu, and truly be present to enjoy the experience of eating. Over time, you'll be amazed at the difference it makes in both the quantity and the quality of what you choose to eat.

Keeping Track

This week, make a commitment to trade your "mindless munching" for the defined meals and snacks listed on your menu. Use your menu to check off what you eat, and allow yourself the 20-minute minimum that it takes for your brain to give the "now I'm satisfied" signal to your stomach. Using your menu to self-monitor will help you re-connect with your body's physical hunger/satisfaction signals.

Social Eater

Goal: Balance the pleasure of eating with healthy choices.

Focus on Planning for Social Situations

If you are a social eater, you struggle with a variety of people, places and events that tempt you to eat. Most likely, you find it difficult to say "no" when offered a favorite dish, both because the food is so appetizing and you don't want to hurt anyone's feelings. You love to dine out. In the moment, when everyone else is so spontaneous in their choices, you follow their lead, and you end up eating not what you'd planned on. And no matter where you go, it seems like portions are huge, but everyone else is eating them, so you do, too. You are committed to your weight loss goals, but you also don't want to deprive yourself the pleasure of dining out, entertaining and spending time with others. Not to worry – you can do both. It just takes some skills, strategies and information to navigate your way past the super-size portions and hidden calories you'll find in many restaurant offerings.

Mastering Social Eating

In your consultations, you'll learn strategies for making smart restaurant selections, as well as secrets to enjoying social situations without feeling left out. Your *Dining Out Success Guide* is filled with information on how/what to eat in a variety of fast food/sit-down restaurants, even if all the nutrition facts are not available. It also includes information on how to include an occasional "splurge". Also, your Jenny Craig cookbooks are a wonderful resource for preparing meals that you can share and enjoy with others as you are losing weight on the program.

Keeping Track

Let your consultant know when you have a social situation coming up and he/she will show you how to use the Meal on My Own servings on your menu to plan for the occasion. Also, use the "Visual Cues for Serving Sizes" on Jenny's Grocery List to keep restaurant portions within your control.

Balanced Eater

Goal: Maintain your healthy relationship with food.

Focus on Maintaining Balanced Eating

Congratulations! You have a healthy relationship with food. You are able to make nutritious choices and balance them with the pleasure of eating.

Mastering Balanced Eating

Throughout the program we will continue to reinforce your healthy relationship with food with the portion control, variety and convenience of Jenny's Cuisine. You will also have the opportunity to focus on other areas of weight management related to Body and Mind – such as increasing your physical activity and fostering a healthy mindset.

Keeping Track

Research repeatedly has shown that self-monitoring, whether in a log, a journal or even in your head, is a key factor in weight loss and weight maintenance. Your Jenny Craig Menu is designed to make self-monitoring quick and easy. Use your menu to cross off the foods you've eaten, circle the ones you haven't, and even write in the extra foods you hadn't planned to eat, but did.

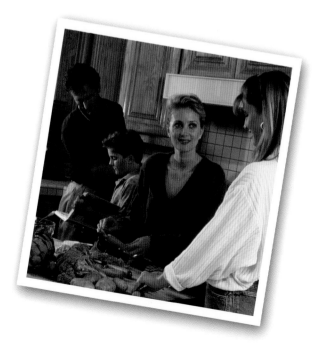

Your Lifestyle
Dining Out and Cooking at Home

For consistent weight loss, plan non-Jenny's Cuisine meals in advance with your consultant. If you can't plan ahead, try this "healthy plate" strategy to help keep you on track:

Fill ½ your plate with vegetables (1-2 cups), ¼ of your plate with starches (½-1 cup) and ¼ of your plate with meat (3-4 ounces).

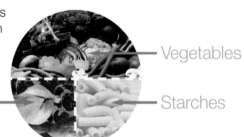

Vegetables

Meat

Starches

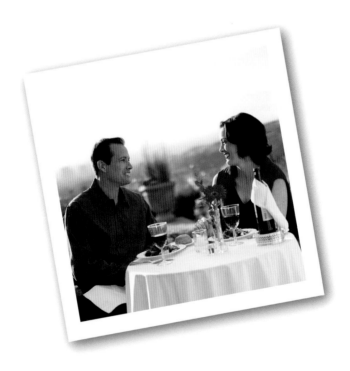

If You Dine Out
Did you know…
According to the National Weight Registry, successful weight maintainers dine out an average of 3.5 times per week, including one time per week at a fast food restaurant.

For more consistent weight loss, you will want to limit dining out, and when you do dine out, rely on your Menu's "Meal on My Own" as a model.

As you progress through your program and begin to plan more meals on your own into your Menu, you will find that the *Jenny Craig Dining Out Success Guide* is a great resource to help you.

If You Cook
If you regularly cook for yourself or others, you'll find our *30 Meals in 30 Minutes Cookbook* and *The Volumetrics® Cookbook for Jenny Craig* great resources for preparing quick and healthy recipes.

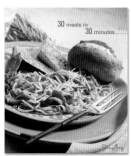

If You Travel
If you frequently travel, you'll want to plan your Menu around portable items from our full line of shelf-stable, microwavable meals, such as Turkey Chili and Chicken Pasta Parmesan. Throw in our other portable items like our Honey Oat Bar or our Chicken and Tuna Salad Kits and Trail Mix and you have everything you need for a program on-the-go. All of our travel-friendly foods are denoted by a 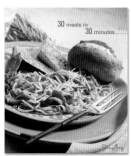 on your Menu Planner.

Body

Dispelling the Myths

Now that you've gotten on track with your menu, it's time to explore the other half of the energy balance equation: physical activity. Let's start by dispelling the common myths...

Myth: I can turn fat into muscle.
Fact: Fat and muscle are distinct tissues. The only way to positively change your body composition is to lose fat by burning calories and gain muscle by engaging in resistance activity.

Myth: I might get bulky if I lift weights.
Fact: If your goal is to tone and get a leaner body, lifting lighter weights at higher repetitions will help you. The only way you'll develop big muscles is if you participate in intensive training and lift heavy weights at fewer repetitions. Women have less testosterone hormone than men and are less likely to get bulky muscles. Strength training can lead to more muscle definition, tone, strength and increased bone density, which will reduce the risk of osteoporosis. And, as we've mentioned, increased muscle mass will lead to a higher metabolism.

Myth: I can spot reduce to lose weight from my thighs.
Fact: Spot reducing is a myth; spot toning isn't. Cardio activities such as biking and running help burn overall body fat. Resistance activities such as yoga or lifting weights can tone and improve the appearance of individual muscles, such as those in the thighs.

Myth: It's better to be apple-shaped than pear-shaped.
Fact: People who carry most of their excess weight around the waist (apple shape) are at greater risk for diabetes and heart disease than those who carry most of their excess weight below the waist (pear shape). The good news is that you can lower your risk of these conditions by losing as little as 5-10% of your start weight, no matter what shape you are.

Myth: It's better to exercise in the morning than in the evening.
Fact: Some people prefer morning workouts to start off their day. Others use afternoon or evening workouts for stress-relief. Some research has shown that morning exercisers are more likely to stay in the habit, while

other research has shown that the muscles are warmer and looser in the afternoon, leading to higher exercise performance and reduced injury. The one thing that everyone agrees on is that developing a routine to fit your lifestyle and one you are likely to stay with is the most important thing. The best time to exercise is the time that works for you. No matter what time of day it is, physical activity will burn calories, reduce stress and enhance your mood. If you find that a morning workout fits into your schedule the best, just spend a few more minutes warming up and stretching.

Myth: I need to eat extra protein to build muscle.
Fact: Excess protein is not stored as muscle. In fact, extra calories from protein, fat or carbohydrates can result in weight gain. The Jenny Craig Program is designed to provide 20-30% of your calories as protein, which is more than adequate to meet the requirements of most athletes. Your menu calorie level was tailored to provide adequate nutrition for the amount of activity you were doing when you started the program. If your activity level greatly increases during the program, speak with your consultant about re-evaluating your calorie level as necessary.

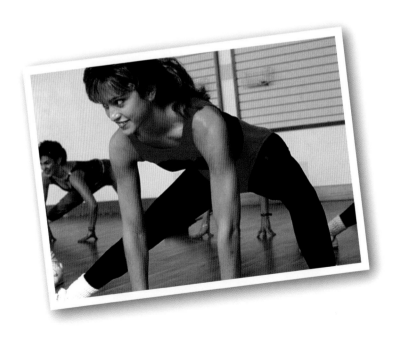

The Value Of An Active Lifestyle

During the third week of your program, you will begin to focus on the second success factor for reaching your weight loss goals – the Body, or active lifestyle component of the program.

Research has shown that an active lifestyle is a critical factor in successful weight loss. While it's true that physical activity supports consistent weight loss, its role is even more critical in long-term weight maintenance. In research conducted by the National Weight Control Registry of 4500 individuals who have lost at least 30 lbs. and kept it off for 1 year, it was found that, on average, these individuals are physically active for 60 minutes a day. The good news is, the "exercise" is a combination of walking, resistance and "natural" activity. The bottom line: it's not a strenuous exercise regimen, but an active lifestyle that makes the difference between maintainers and weight re-gainers. At Jenny Craig, you'll learn strategies for building the active lifestyle to enhance your own success.

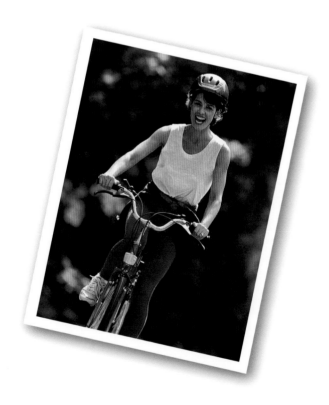

Setting Up Your Activity Plan

To set up your activity plan, you'll want to start by identifying three things: your barriers, your benefits and your support system.

Your Barriers and Benefits

It's natural for things to stand in the way of adding activity into your daily routine—especially in our society where cars, escalators, power tools and other labor-saving devices make it easy to be sedentary.

Take a few minutes to list your personal physical activity barriers.

Physical Activity Barriers:

- _____
- _____
- _____
- _____
- _____
- _____
- _____

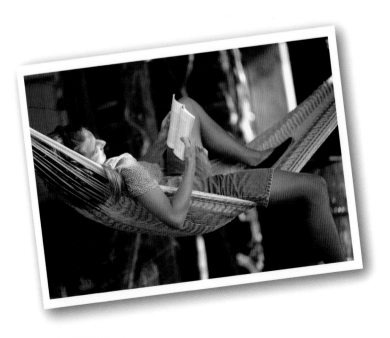

During your consultations, your consultant will work with you to develop plans to overcome your barriers. Another way to motivate yourself to get over the barriers is to get creative with your solutions and remind yourself of all the benefits you can get from being active. Here are a few that may be of interest to you...

Name your physical activity benefits:

☐ 1. Burns calories for weight loss

☐ 2. Increases energy

☐ 3. Decreases stress

☐ 4. Maintains muscle mass and metabolism

☐ 5. Improves self-confidence

☐ 6. Is a success factor for weight maintenance

☐ 7. Lowers the risk for heart disease

☐ 8. Improves diabetes control

☐ 9. Lowers the risk of developing osteoporosis

☐ 10. Lowers the risk for some types of cancers

☐ Other:_____

_____

Reviewing the list above, check off the benefits you look forward to enjoying by increasing your physical activity. Or, if there are other benefits not listed above, write them in, so you can refer to them as well.

As you progress through your program, you will want to return to this page often and cross out the barriers you've overcome and add the new benefits you've discovered. The fewer barriers you have, the easier it will be to achieve and enjoy a more active lifestyle.

Blair SN, Dunn AL, Marcus BH, et al. *Active Living Every Day: 20 Steps to Lifelong Vitality*. Champaign, IL: Human Kinetics, 2001.

Your Support System

Studies have shown that having the support of others can help you reach your weight loss goals. At Jenny Craig, your consultant is always here to support you, but what about your friends and family members? They are probably more than willing to help, and all you need to do is ask.

Use the form below to help you identify people who can support your physical activity efforts. Fill in the boxes under "What do I need help with?" Then, think about the best people to turn to for the specific help you need. After you've identified your best supporters, all you need to do is ask for their support in reaching your goals.

My Support Troops

What do I need help with?
Who could help me?
How could they help?
How could I reward them for helping me?

Blair SN, Dunn AL, Marcus BH, et al. *Active Living Every Day: 20 Steps to Lifelong Vitality*. Champaign, IL: Human Kinetics, 2001.

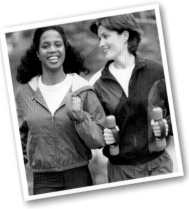

Get Ready to Move!

Ask weight loss clients why they exercise, and often they'll tell you it's to burn calories. Ask weight maintenance clients why, and it could be for the energy, pleasure and self-confidence they feel when they're regularly active. In fact, physical activity has become a part of their lifestyle. That's great, because physical activity is the number one success factor for weight maintenance.

Where to Start

How did the weight maintainer get to that point? In stages—from just thinking about being active, to getting ready to be active, to being and then staying active. That's what this portion of your program is about—a personalized, staged approach that starts where you are right now and builds from there. Where to begin? **Your**Style® Profile tells us what stage you were in when you began the program. As you progress through the program we will return to the Personal Activity Quiz on the following page to re-check your stage and continue to tailor your activities.

How to Track

Use the Body section on the front of your menu to:
- Record your "Activity Plan for the Week".
  This will help you stay focused on your goal.
- Track your "Activity/Time/Steps" each day.
  This will help you track your progress and set new goals.
- Note your "Pre and Post Activity Feelings".
  This will motivate you to move more!

- ***Notice*** *the increase in your energy, clarity and relaxation.*
- ***Focus*** *on how good it feels to move your body through space.*
- ***Visualize*** *your muscles getting stronger and more fit.*
- ***Challenge*** *the perception of exercise as "work."*
- ***Feel*** *the empowerment of your healthy changes.*

A Special Note

Be sure to discuss your activity goals with your physician, especially if you are older then 40, smoke, have pulmonary disease, high blood pressure, diabetes or musculoskeletal disease.

Personal Activity Quiz *(check the boxes that apply to you)*

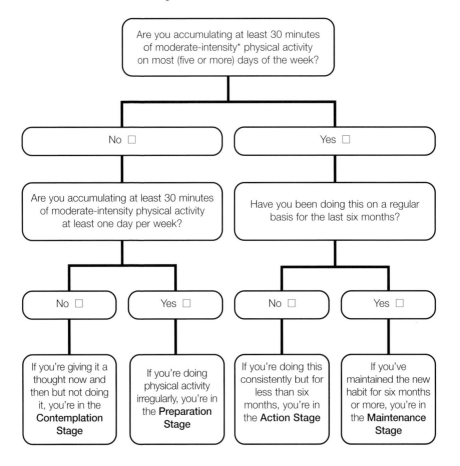

Are you accumulating at least 30 minutes of moderate-intensity* physical activity on most (five or more) days of the week?

No ☐

Yes ☐

Are you accumulating at least 30 minutes of moderate-intensity physical activity at least one day per week?

Have you been doing this on a regular basis for the last six months?

No ☐   Yes ☐   No ☐   Yes ☐

If you're giving it a thought now and then but not doing it, you're in the **Contemplation Stage**

If you're doing physical activity irregularly, you're in the **Preparation Stage**

If you're doing this consistently but for less than six months, you're in the **Action Stage**

If you've maintained the new habit for six months or more, you're in the **Maintenance Stage**

---

*Moderate-intensity physical activities are equal in effort to a brisk walk, walking a mile in 15 to 20 minutes. Here are examples of other moderate-intensity activities:

- Bicycling (10-12 mph)
- Dancing
- Gardening and doing yard work
- Golfing (without a cart)
- Hiking

- Playing actively with children
- Raking leaves
- Vacuuming a carpet
- Playing volleyball
- Hand-washing and waxing a car

Blair SN, Dunn AL, Marcus BH, et al. *Active Living Every Day: 20 Steps to Lifelong Vitality*. Champaign, IL: Human Kinetics, 2001.

What's Your Activity Stage?

Learn more about your Activity Stage by referring to the section that corresponds to YourStyle® profile results...

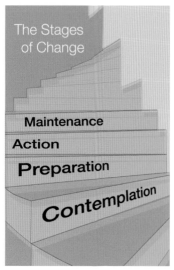

The Stages of Change

Maintenance

Action

Preparation

Contemplation

Contemplation – thinking about it
- Beginning to think about including more activity in your lifestyle, but not yet being active. See page 37.

Preparation – getting ready to do it
- Accumulating at least 30 minutes of moderate-intensity activity at least one day per week, but not on most days of the week. See page 41.

Action – doing it
- Accumulating at least 30 minutes of moderate-intensity activity on five or more days of the week, but have done so for less than six months. See page 48.

Maintenance – have been doing it
- Accumulating at least 30 minutes of moderate-intensity activity on five or more days a week for six months or more. See page 52.

Know that you won't always progress directly from one stage to the next one. You may begin at Preparation and then move back into Contemplation before progressing to Action. That's the nature of change. Everyone is unique and will progress through the stages differently. The key is that you are trying to make a change.

The activities in this book are adapted from <u>Active Living Every Day</u>, *which was developed by Human Kinetics and The Cooper Institute.* <u>Active Living Every Day</u> *is a behavior change program designed to help inactive people become and stay physically active for a lifetime. Jenny Craig supports this stage-based approach to physical activity. To learn more, please visit their Web site at www.activeliving.info.*

The Stages

Contemplation

Goal: Move to Preparation stage and incorporate small amounts of physical activity.

Focus on Natural Activity

Don't have time to exercise? Think you don't know how to exercise? Relax, the goal is simple: just move a little more today than yesterday. That's really all it takes to get started. And the best way to achieve this is to incorporate activity into your everyday routine.

When people think about exercise, they envision long, strenuous workouts. The truth is that exercise ranges from walking to the neighbor's house to gardening to running a marathon. Every move you make—hand-washing the car, vacuuming the house, walking the dog—counts.

As you begin to lose weight and your fitness level increases from more activity, you can ease into moderately intense activities such as brisk walking. What does brisk mean? Think of it as a late-to-a-meeting walk. Technically, it means walking a mile in 15-20 minutes. For now, the best goal you can set is to simply incorporate more natural activity into your daily routine. **To keep track of your natural activity, add up your minutes in the "Body" section of your menu.** You'll be surprised how quickly they add up.

Look at the calories you can burn from everyday activities.

Natural Activity	Calories/1 minute				
	140 lbs.	180 lbs.	200 lbs.	240 lbs.	260 lbs.
Cleaning, light	2.8	3.6	4.0	4.8	5.2
Cooking	2.2	2.9	3.2	3.8	4.1
Playing Catch	2.8	3.6	4.0	4.8	5.2
Shopping	2.6	3.3	3.7	4.4	4.7
Washing Dishes	2.6	3.3	3.7	4.4	4.7

Blair SN, Dunn AL, Marcus BH, et al. *Active Living Every Day: 20 Steps to Lifelong Vitality*. Champaign, IL: Human Kinetics, 2001:179-182.

Mastering Contemplation

Opportunities to Move

One of the main barriers to an active lifestyle, and probably one you included on your list of barriers, is time. Everyone is busy. But do you know where all the minutes in the day go? How much time do you spend at the computer, watching TV, etc? It's helpful to take a look at how you spend your time. This can help you identify opportunities for activity that you might not have been aware of—like walking around during your child's baseball game, vigorously vacuuming during the TV commercials or going for a 15-minute walk at lunch. The "Personal Time Study" on the next two pages will help you identify times in your day where you can include activity.

Learn about yourself

On the next two pages record your activities for one week day and one weekend day. Use the sheets provided or use a notepad if your prefer. Keep the record with you and write things down as you go. Remember to add up the minutes you were physically active and record those in the "Yes" column. Then add up the minutes you were inactive and record those in the "No" column. The total active and inactive time for each four-hour block should be 240 minutes. Add up the total number of active and inactive minutes in your day at the bottom of the sheet.

EXAMPLE:

Time Slot	Tasks and activities	Physically active?	
		Yes	No
8:01 A.M. to noon	Walk to and from car:	7 minutes	
	Desk work:		75 minutes
	Meeting:		120 minutes
	Walk to vending machine:	3 minutes	
	Walk to meeting:	4 minutes	
	Talk with coworkers:		31 minutes
Total time:		14 minutes	226 minutes
12:01 P.M. 4:00 P.M.	Walk to lunch room:	5 minutes	
	Lunch:		30 minutes
	Walk back to office:	5 minutes	
	Desk work:		180 minutes
	Walk to lunch room:	5 minutes	
	Coffee break:		10 minutes
	Return to office:	5 minutes	
Total time:		20 minutes	220 minutes

Personal Time Study

Date: _____

Day of week: _____

Time Slot	Tasks and activities	Physically active?	
		Yes	No
Midnight to 4:00 A.M.			
4:01 A.M. to 8:00 A.M.			
8:01 A.M. to noon			
12:01 P.M. to 4:00 P.M.			
4:01 P.M. to 8:00 P.M.			
8:01 P.M. to midnight			
	Total time		

Did you find opportunities to incorporate more
physical activity into your lifestyle?

Blair SN, Dunn AL, Marcus BH, et al. *Active Living Every Day: 20 Steps to Lifelong Vitality*. Champaign, IL: Human Kinetics, 2001.

Keeping Track

People who track their activities by keeping a log are more successful at changing habits than those who don't. Because you are not yet regularly active, it will be helpful for you to just keep track of the time you think about doing activity on the form below. Chances are, the more you find yourself thinking about activity the sooner you'll be ready to take action.

Keeping Track of Thoughts

Week of: _____

Instructions: Use this section to record the number of times you think about doing some physical activity. Simply place a check mark ✔ in a box in section 1 each time you *think* about doing some physical activity. If you carried out your thoughts and did the activity you were thinking about, place a check mark ✔ in a box in section 2.

Section 1.

I thought about doing some physical activity.

Section 2.

I carried out the thoughts and did the activity.

Keep this form handy so you can record your thoughts about physical activity whenever they occur!

Blair SN, Dunn AL, Marcus BH, et al. *Active Living Every Day: 20 Steps to Lifelong Vitality*. Champaign, IL: Human Kinetics, 2001.

Preparation

Goal: Move to Action stage and accumulate at least 30 minutes of moderate-intensity activity on five or more days a week.

Focus on Playful Activity

When you're juggling multiple priorities, it's easy to put activity on the bottom of the list. Playful activities give permission for you to take the time to be active, without taking quality time away from family and friends. Join your kids for tag or basketball. Instead of going to a movie with friends, go dancing.

The best way to be active is to feel like you're playing and having fun. And just look at the calories you can burn while you're doing it!

Playful activity	140 lbs.	180 lbs.	Calories/1 minute 200 lbs.	240 lbs.	260 lbs.
Dancing	5.0	6.5	7.2	8.6	9.3
Golfing	5.0	6.5	7.2	8.6	9.3
Bicycling, 10mph	4.5	5.7	6.4	7.6	8.3
Fishing	3.9	5.0	5.6	6.7	7.2
Swimming, leisure	6.7	8.6	9.6	11.4	12.4

Blair SN, Dunn AL, Marcus BH, et al. *Active Living Every Day: 20 Steps to Lifelong Vitality*. Champaign, IL: Human Kinetics, 2001:179-182.

Mastering Preparation

Goal Setting

Experts have found that setting goals is one of the most important keys to success. You identified a short-term and a long-term weight loss goal at the beginning of your program. Now that you are beginning to incorporate more activity into your lifestyle, it is a great time to set specific activity goals.

• The more specific and clear your goal, the more likely you are to reach it.
• It's important to set short-term goals on the way to achieving the long-term goal.

> **Short-term goal** – *increase my steps by 500 per day for the next two weeks*
>
> **Long-term goal** – *increase my steps to 10,000 per day*

• You have options to track your progress. **You may want to count your steps by using our Calorie Walk Pedometer (see page 46), or add up the time you spend performing activities and record your minutes on your menu.**

Use the following form to set a goal you intend to meet.

Ready? Set? Goals!

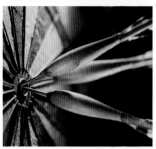

Good goals are...
- ✔ Specific   ✔ Attainable
- ✔ Measurable   ✔ Realistic

A short-term goal I can achieve in the next week:

_____

_____

_____

_____

How I plan to monitor my progress:

☐ Calorie Walk

☐ Minutes on menu

☐ Other _____

_____

A long-term goal I hope to achieve by _____(date):

_____

_____

_____

_____

Post your goals where you'll see them often (for example, on your daily calendar, dresser or bathroom mirror).

Blair SN, Dunn AL, Marcus BH, et al. *Active Living Every Day: 20 Steps to Lifelong Vitality*. Champaign, IL: Human Kinetics, 2001.

Rewards

Now that you've set both your short-term and long-term goals, it's time to think about how you'll reward yourself for reaching your goals.

In studies done at The Cooper Institute and Brown University, people who increased their use of rewards were far more likely to remain active over time than those who didn't give themselves rewards. But, how do you reward yourself?

What about: *A massage, a manicure, a new book or music CD, a bouquet of flowers, a round of golf or an afternoon to yourself?*

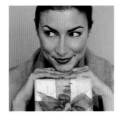

Identifying Rewards

Make a list of ways you can reward yourself for achieving your short-term goals. These should be simple, small rewards.

- _____
- _____
- _____
- _____
- _____
- _____

Write down ideas for rewards that might help spur you on to reaching your long-term goal. These can be more significant than the rewards for your short-term goals.

- _____
- _____
- _____
- _____
- _____

Blair SN, Dunn AL, Marcus BH, et al. *Active Living Every Day: 20 Steps to Lifelong Vitality*. Champaign, IL: Human Kinetics, 2001.

Now, from your list of rewards, choose at least one you'll give yourself for reaching your short-term goal and one for reaching your long-term goal. Write down the goals and the rewards on the "My Contract". Once you've made a contract with yourself, you're far more likely to be committed to reaching your goals.

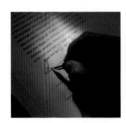

My Contract

When I meet my short-term goal, which is:

_____

I will reward myself with:

_____

When I meet my long-term goal, which is:

_____,

I will reward myself with:

_____

Blair SN, Dunn AL, Marcus BH, et al. *Active Living Every Day: 20 Steps to Lifelong Vitality*. Champaign, IL: Human Kinetics, 2001.

Keeping Track

You have options to track your progress. You may want to count your steps/calories by using your pedometer when walking, or add up the minutes you spend performing other activities. Either way, record your results on your menu.

Keeping Track of Physical Activity

Week of: _____

Instructions: This form is for you to check the amount of time you spend on various activities. After doing an activity, mark the box that best describes the intensity of your activity, moderate or vigorous (see examples below), and its duration. At the end of your week, add the number of minutes checked for each activity category and place it in the "Total" column.

ACTIVITY	LEVEL	2 MINUTES	10 MINUTES	TOTAL
Garden	Moderate	☐☐☐☐☐ ☐☐☐☐☐ ☐☐☐☐☐	☐☐☐☐☐ ☐☐☐☐☐ ☐☐☐☐☐	
	Vigorous	☐☐☐☐☐ ☐☐☐☐☐ ☐☐☐☐☐	☐☐☐☐☐ ☐☐☐☐☐ ☐☐☐☐☐	
Household	Moderate	☐☐☐☐☐ ☐☐☐☐☐ ☐☐☐☐☐	☐☐☐☐☐ ☐☐☐☐☐ ☐☐☐☐☐	
	Vigorous	☐☐☐☐☐ ☐☐☐☐☐ ☐☐☐☐☐	☐☐☐☐☐ ☐☐☐☐☐ ☐☐☐☐☐	
Leisure	Moderate	☐☐☐☐☐ ☐☐☐☐☐ ☐☐☐☐☐	☐☐☐☐☐ ☐☐☐☐☐ ☐☐☐☐☐	
	Vigorous	☐☐☐☐☐ ☐☐☐☐☐ ☐☐☐☐☐	☐☐☐☐☐ ☐☐☐☐☐ ☐☐☐☐☐	
Occupation	Moderate	☐☐☐☐☐ ☐☐☐☐☐ ☐☐☐☐☐	☐☐☐☐☐ ☐☐☐☐☐ ☐☐☐☐☐	
	Vigorous	☐☐☐☐☐ ☐☐☐☐☐ ☐☐☐☐☐	☐☐☐☐☐ ☐☐☐☐☐ ☐☐☐☐☐	
Sports	Moderate	☐☐☐☐☐ ☐☐☐☐☐ ☐☐☐☐☐	☐☐☐☐☐ ☐☐☐☐☐ ☐☐☐☐☐	
	Vigorous	☐☐☐☐☐ ☐☐☐☐☐ ☐☐☐☐☐	☐☐☐☐☐ ☐☐☐☐☐ ☐☐☐☐☐	
Stairs 1 flight up = 10 steps	Vigorous (4 flights up = 2 minutes vigorous work)	☐☐☐☐☐ ☐☐☐☐☐ ☐☐☐☐☐ ☐☐☐☐☐	☐☐☐☐☐ ☐☐☐☐☐ ☐☐☐☐☐ ☐☐☐☐☐	
Walking	Moderate	☐☐☐☐☐ ☐☐☐☐☐ ☐☐☐☐☐	☐☐☐☐☐ ☐☐☐☐☐ ☐☐☐☐☐	
	Vigorous	☐☐☐☐☐ ☐☐☐☐☐ ☐☐☐☐☐	☐☐☐☐☐ ☐☐☐☐☐ ☐☐☐☐☐	

Example of Activities

Activity	Moderate	Vigorous (hard or very hard)
Garden	Raking, mowing (push), weeding	Shoveling, carrying moderate/heavy loads
Household	Vacuuming carpet, cleaning windows	Moving furniture, shoveling snow
Leisure	Ballroom dancing, fishing from bank (standing or wading)	Pop dancing, backpacking
Occupation	Walking briskly at work	Using heavy tools, firefighting, loading/unloading truck, laying brick
Sports	Table tennis, golf (no cart), tai chi, Frisbee	Rope jumping, basketball, running, racquetball, soccer
Walking	15-20 minute/mile (1.6 km) pace	Stair climbing, mountain biking

Blair SN, Dunn AL, Marcus BH, et al. *Active Living Every Day: 20 Steps to Lifelong Vitality*. Champaign, IL: Human Kinetics, 2001.

Jenny Craig Tools

Jenny Craig Pedometer

Walking is one of the easiest ways to incorporate activity into your daily routine, but can be difficult to monitor. One way to keep track of your walking is by using a pedometer. This tiny tool clips to your belt and registers each step you take (every 2,000 steps equals approximately one mile).

How to use the pedometer:
- Simply clip it to your belt just over your hip when you get dressed in the morning.
- Set it to zero.
- Take the pedometer off before going to bed at night and record the number of steps for the day. Do this for seven days.
- Continue your current activity for the first week. This will tell you how many steps per day you usually get.
- After that, start adding steps. A good initial goal is to aim for 2000 additional steps in your day.

Our pedometer is a great way to not only monitor your steps, but to track the calories you've burned, and to help you set your "stretch" goals. Remember, it takes a deficit of 3500 calories to lose a pound. Why not aim for the number of steps that burns an additional 250 calories per day? This will lead to an additional half pound of weight loss per week, without having to decrease your calorie intake. As you can see, the more activity you can fit into your day, the more flexibility you'll have with your food intake, especially at maintenance.

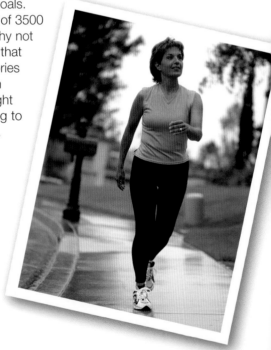

For health benefits, a good goal is to walk at least 10,000 steps every day. Try for even more steps on the weekends, vacations or holidays when you have a bit more time.

In addition to tracking your steps and helping you set goals, the pedometer is also a great motivator. You can take the dog for a walk and walk to a friend's house instead of driving and see your steps increasing on your pedometer. Seeing how your daily activities add up and knowing that each one contributes to your calories burned for weight loss can inspire you to set even higher goals.

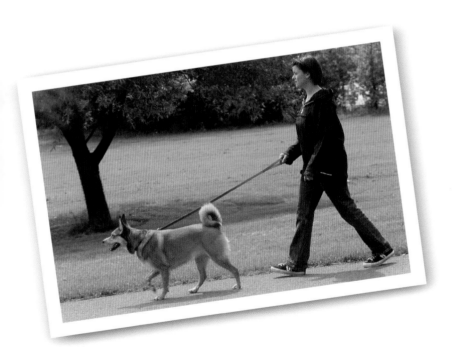

Action

Goal: Move to Maintenance stage and accumulate at least 30 minutes of moderate- to high-intensity activity on five or more days a week, for six months or more.

Focus on Planned Activity

You're doing a great job being regularly active. Now is a good time to begin adding some new activities. If you've focused primarily on moderate-intensity activities like walking or biking, why not boost your metabolism with resistance training? If you're already doing both, focus on the mind/body benefits of stretching activities like yoga. Yoga offers a combination of resistance and stretching that can be both energizing and relaxing.

The best activity plan for weight loss and maintenance includes cardio, resistance and stretching. **Remember to use the "Body" section of your menu to record your minutes of each type of activity.**

Cardio
What counts as cardio activity? Any activity that burns calories and strengthens the heart. Whether you choose to walk, bike, or do the stair climber remember the components of the ideal workout:

Warm up (5-10 minutes) – prepares your muscles to move and minimizes your risk for injury

Cardio (30-60 minutes) – burns calories and strengthens your heart

Cool down (5-10 minutes) – relaxes your muscles and brings your heart rate back to normal

See page 49 for ideas for adding cardio to your weekly activity plan.

Resistance
For every pound of muscle you gain, your body expends an additional 20-45 calories per day. Sit-ups, push-ups and exercises using light weights will improve the physical appearance of muscles without greatly increasing their size or bulk. Start with 10 minutes of floor work or light weights.

Stretching
Stretching prevents injury, enhances flexibility and rejuvenates your body and mind. Listen to your body. Avoid bouncing or jerking movements and focus on holding a stretch for 10-30 seconds. To avoid injury stretch only to the point of mild tension.

Planned Activity	Calories/1 minute				
	140 lbs.	180 lbs.	200 lbs.	240 lbs.	260 lbs.
Weightlifting, vigorous effort	6.7	8.6	9.6	11.4	12.4
Walking 20 min per mile	3.7	4.7	5.3	6.3	6.8
Aerobic dance, low impact	5.6	7.2	8.0	9.5	10.3
Stair climber	10.1	12.9	14.3	17.2	18.6
Running 8 min per mile	14.0	17.9	19.9	23.8	25.8
Step aerobics, 6" to 8" step	9.5	12.2	13.5	16.2	17.6
Judo, karate, kickboxing	11.2	14.4	15.9	19.1	20.7
Bicycling, 12-12mph	9.0	11.5	12.7	15.3	16.5

Blair SN, Dunn AL, Marcus BH, et al. *Active Living Every Day: 20 Steps to Lifelong Vitality*. Champaign, IL: Human Kinetics, 2001:179-182.

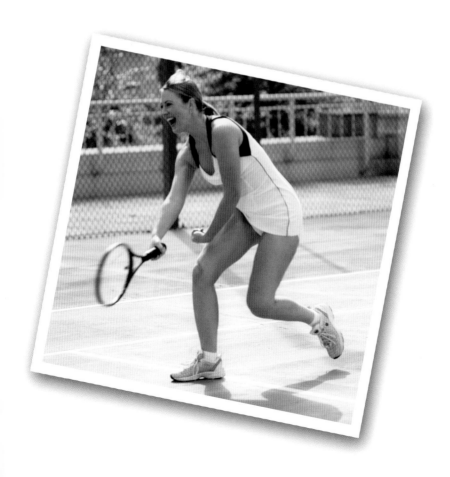

Mastering Action

Now is also a good time to investigate new places to be active—to keep your routine fresh and provide options for a busy lifestyle.

New Opportunities to Be Active

Use this form to keep track of opportunities you find in your community for physical activity. As you fill in this form, think about the new physical activities or opportunities you'd like to learn more about. Place a star by your top two and give them a try.

Parks	Location	Comments
Recreation Centers	**Location**	**Comments**
Activity Clubs	**Location**	**Comments**
Other		

Blair SN, Dunn AL, Marcus BH, et al. *Active Living Every Day*: 20 Steps to Lifelong Vitality. Champaign, IL: Human Kinetics, 2001.

Rewards

One way to help you stay on track and remain consistent with your activity is to make sure you're rewarding yourself. If you've already established your personal rewards in the Preparation stage, now is a good time to revisit them and see if you want to make any changes. Maybe you'd like a new outfit or a CD to listen to while you walk. See page 43 to make a list of ways you can reward yourself, or to review the list you've already created.

Jenny Craig Tools

Resistance Cord Kit

Looking for a way to add a resistant component to your activity routine? Want to tone your muscles without having to lift weights or go to the gym? The Gaiam Resistance Cord Kit is a complete portable resistance training system that allows you to work out anywhere, anytime and add a resistance component to your routine. This great tool will help you improve your total body tone and flexibility.

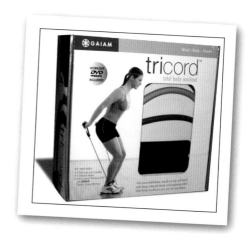

The kit features:
• Three levels of intensity
• An expert-guided DVD workout (60 min)

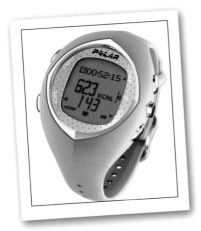

Calorie and Heart Rate Monitor

Want to safely increase the intensity or calories burned during your activity? The Polar Calorie and Heart Rate Monitor accurately measures calories burned while ensuring that you stay in a safe, effective and sustainable heart rate zone. It also measures activities that can't be measured by a pedometer, like swimming, biking or resistance training.

Functions include:
• Calories burned during any physical activity
• Recommended heart rate and target heart rate zone
• Total minutes and average heart rate of activity
• Visible and audible target zone alarm to stay within a safe zone
• Time of day
• Stopwatch

Maintenance

Goal: Stay in the Maintenance stage. What an accomplishment! You've maintained an active lifestyle for six months or more.

Focus on Maintenance

Where Do You Go From Here?

It's true that at least 30 minutes of moderate-intensity activity on most days is enough to reap health benefits. However, research by the National Weight Control Registry suggests that, for weight maintenance, more activity may be better. In a study of 2800 individuals who kept off at least 30 pounds for more than five years, the average weekly activity level added up to 2800 calories, the equivalent of one hour of activity per day. The great news is, these active individuals don't exercise daily to exhaustion. They've threaded activity into their days. They engage in a near-equal mix of natural and cardio activity (primarily walking) and many have made resistance activity a habit, as well.

The Maintenance stage is the perfect time to push a little harder, set some new goals and renew your commitment. Doing so will help you to stay with all the healthy changes you have made so far.

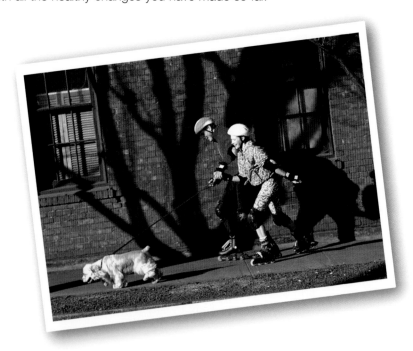

Mastering Maintenance

My Plan to Push a Little Harder

1. Do you plan to increase or maintain your current activity level?
   Circle one: Increase   Maintain

2. If you are planning to increase your physical activity level, circle the
   things you plan to increase:

   Frequency   Types of activities   Intensity   Amount of time (duration)

3. Now list the strategies you will use to put your plan into action.
   Be specific. (Check all that apply).

   ☐ Set new short-term goal(s):

   _____

   ☐ Reward myself with _____
      for meeting my short-term goal.

   ☐ Set new long-term goal(s):

   _____

   ☐ Reward myself with _____
      for meeting my long-term goal.

   ☐ Self-monitor using either a step counter or by keeping track of
      minutes on my menu. Circle one: Calorie Walk   Minutes

   ☐ Enlist my support troops:

   _____

   ☐ Try a new activity:

   _____

   ☐ Plan for high-risk situations: (These are places, events, times or
      people that may sidetrack your physical activity efforts. Holidays, illness
      and busy times at work are common high-risk situations).

   _____

   _____

Blair SN, Dunn AL, Marcus BH, et al. *Active Living Every Day: 20 Steps to Lifelong Vitality*. Champaign, IL: Human Kinetics, 2001.

Mind

Dispelling the Myths

Just as there are many myths out there related to Food and Body, you may have heard some of the following myths related to the Mind aspect of weight loss...

Myth: With all the family/work demands on my schedule, there isn't always enough time for a weight loss program.
Fact: Although lifestyle change requires energy, it can also give you energy. As you go through the process, you'll begin to create a healthier life balance. You'll feel less overwhelmed and more resourceful and available to others. The convenience of the Jenny Craig Program and menu can help you save time and practice self-care when things are hectic.

Myth: To lose weight, I have to follow a diet perfectly.
Fact: Weight loss is about progress, not perfection. In fact, a study of Jenny Craig clients demonstrates just that. Those clients who attended at least 12 of their first 16 weekly consultations lost an average of 17.5 pounds, or 8.9% of their starting weight. That's an amount that health experts say can help lower the risk for heart disease, high blood pressure and diabetes.

Myth: Once the program ends, I can go back to a "normal" life.
Fact: Any effective weight loss program should be designed to help you establish healthy habits that you can maintain for a lifetime. The Jenny Craig Program is not a "crash diet" but a program designed to promote long-term weight management solutions. As you progress through the program, a healthier lifestyle will become the norm for you.

Myth: Losing weight means deprivation.
Fact: Long-term weight loss is achieved with balance and moderation, not deprivation. You are less likely to stay on a program that requires you to give up your favorite things. So, include your favorite foods and give yourself rewards – you are demonstrating a healthy balance, not a lack of willpower.

Myth: Having a lapse is a sign that I can't do this.
Fact: You're learning to lose weight in the real world, not the perfect one. A lapse is not a sign of failure. It is a normal part of the weight loss process. Think of a lapse as an opportunity to build new skills for the future.

Myth: Once I lose weight, my whole life will be different.
Fact: People who successfully lose weight often do change many aspects of their lives. Losing weight will probably change your looks and improve your health and self-confidence. But keep in mind, your body is only one aspect of you as a person. If you have other personal goals for yourself, don't put them on hold until you are finished losing weight, start working toward them now.

The Value of a Healthy Weight Loss Mindset

Successful weight management depends on more than just balancing healthy eating with consistent physical activity. It requires the skills, strategies, information and the *motivation* to maintain positive changes for life.

Motivation is affected by the beliefs and habits you hold about food, your body and even your weight loss efforts. Where did you get those beliefs and behaviors? You learned them from your family, school, the media, even your own values and life experience. Some of these beliefs serve your weight loss efforts, and some don't. Together these beliefs make up a weight loss mindset that can strengthen or sabotage your results.

During your program, you'll explore some of the most common negative beliefs, or mindsets, that can trip up a weight manager's efforts. Think of these mindsets as mental roadblocks. Explore them without judgment. Then move past them, onward to a more positive mindset – one that can be the foundation for all the healthy changes you'll make in your eating style and activity stage. That mindset is the central point that keeps your weight and lifestyle in balance.

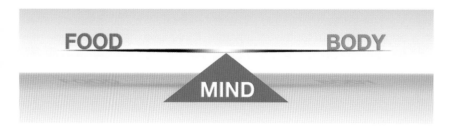

Setting Up Your Mindset

Trade In a Diet for a Lifestyle

When you chose Jenny Craig's **Your**Style®, you chose lifestyle change. That's different from a diet that promises a quick fix, but doesn't give real results. Experts say it's lifestyle change, not diets, that works over the long haul!

Diets Vs.	Lifestyle	The "Lifestyle" Advantage
Self-control	Self-Awareness	Understanding what guides your choices
Deprivation	Moderation	Enjoying all foods in the right portions
Willpower	"Skillpower"	Practicing new habits and healthier thinking
Perfection	Self-Acceptance	Using mistakes as learning opportunities
Radical Change	Real Action	Taking small steps that add up to big results

Set Realistic Weight Expectations

When it comes to losing weight, everyone has a different idea about what to expect. Individual weight loss varies, but here is an overview of the typical pattern:

Phase 1: The Big Drop
Reduce calories, carbohydrates and sodium (salt) during the first week, and your body responds with a typical one to four pound weight loss. This may be exciting and motivating, yet that weight loss is mostly water. Sodium and carbohydrate cause your body to retain fluid, so reducing their intake will have a diuretic (water loss) effect and cause greater initial weight loss.

Phase 2: The Little Drop
In the next week or so, your body begins to burn stored fat. The scale reflects changes in two areas—body fat and water, so you typically see a slightly lower rate of loss, approximately one to three pounds. This is still motivating and absolutely normal. After all, if 50% of your three-pound loss was from fat tissue, that would represent more than 5,000 calories burned in a single week! Aim for this steady rate. If you lose more rapidly, you may lose muscle, which decreases your metabolism and increases your chance of re-gaining weight.

Phase 3: The Slow and Steady

After a few weeks, water loss is complete. That's when you'll see your rate of loss decrease a bit more, usually between one-half and two pounds. Not to worry—you're right where you are supposed to be. The scale is reflecting true weight loss, and that's primarily fat loss! How to know? Along with weekly weights, your monthly measurements—the inches lost—provide the proof. Use your Lifestyle Graph to stay motivated and focus on the big picture: the downward trend in total pounds and inches lost, along with the increase in healthy behaviors and confidence.

What's Your Weight Loss Mindset?

Learn more about your weight loss Mindsets by referring to the sections that correspond to YourStyle® Profile results...

Inner Critic – focusing on your shortcomings
You may be overly critical and judgmental of yourself. See pages 58-59.

Self-Sacrificer- putting everyone else's needs before your own
You may be neglecting yourself. See pages 59-60.

Weight Pessimist – focusing on what didn't work, versus what did.
You may be missing out on all your positive changes. See pages 61-62.

Diet Extremist – taking an all or nothing approach to your weight loss efforts.
You may find it difficult to stay on track with your eating and physical activity plan. See pages 62-63.

Lifestyle Moderate – making small, consistent changes in your food and activity.
Your goal is "progress, not perfection" and you are looking to make realistic changes that you can maintain for life. See page 63.

The Mindsets

Inner-Critic

Goal: Learn to validate yourself.

Focus on Self-Acceptance

Are you a perfectionist? Being a perfectionist isn't about being perfect; it's about being hypercritical and judgmental. For weight managers, it can run the range between minimizing your best efforts and blaming your lapses on character defects or lack of willpower. Interestingly, experts say you're more likely to make positive lifestyle changes if you practice self-acceptance. If you accept yourself, with all your strengths and weaknesses, you can more objectively look at your behaviors, and more clearly make choices to change them.

Mastering Self-Acceptance

It takes time to build your affirming skills. In fact, you'll have the support of your Jenny Craig consultant to help you learn to reframe even the most challenging situations in a more positive light. Lapses happen – it's how you respond to them that matters. Here's a four-step technique that can make the difference in your results.

<u>Four Step Solution</u>

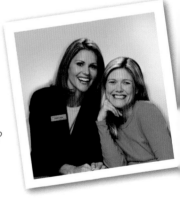

1. Forgive Yourself –
2. Analyze the Situation
   - *Where were you?*
   - *Who was there?*
   - *What was going on?*
   - *What did you feel?*
   - *What did you say to yourself?*
   - *What did you do?*
3. Plan a New Strategy
4. Rehearse, Rehearse, Rehearse

Discuss your plan with your consultant.

Keeping Track

Self-validation may not come easily to you, but that's ok. This week, start practicing self-validation by recording your positive changes or successes as "Wins" on your menu. Your successes do not need to be monumental – they can be as simple as deciding to eat your Jenny's Cuisine lunch when you were feeling tempted to go through the drive-thru. You can get great gratification from just following through on your plan. When you take the walk instead of the cookie, you will feel empowered. Behaving in a way that is consistent with your values and your personal motivators will help you see your program not as a regimen, but as a way to build your self-confidence and self-esteem.

Self-Sacrificer

Goal: Practice self-care.

Focus on Self-Care

As a self-sacrificer, you tend to put everyone else's needs before your own. You juggle multiple roles – parent, spouse, professional, caregiver, volunteer – that frequently overshadow your own personal priorities. As a result, you may pass on your activity plan or use the immediate gratification of food to address stress issues. Experts say that successful weight managers develop a sort of healthy "selfishness" that strikes a balance between being totally self-oriented and overly other-directed. By taking time to relax, re-charge and focus on non-food ways to rejuvenate, self-nurturers build a stress resilience that serves both themselves and others.

Mastering Self-Care

Managing your stress is an important aspect of self-care. Everybody experiences some stress in their daily lives. Stress can come from many sources – your job, your family, a change in plans or an uncomfortable situation. Stress may be part of the reason that you often find it difficult to practice self-care. In fact, some common methods of "coping" with stress - such as using food or alcohol, may actually increase stress and negatively impact your self-care and weight loss goals. Although you can't eliminate stress from your life, there are ways to effectively reduce it and manage it.

In your consultations, you'll identify your mind/body stressors, as well as simple strategies to respond in healthier ways. This week, if you find yourself feeling overwhelmed by the weight of the world, try using your breath to center yourself and quiet your mind.
• Inhale deeply. Feel your abdomen fill with air.
• Hold that breath for a few seconds.
• Slowly exhale, first from the abdomen, and then up through the chest.
• Repeat 5 times.

Keeping Track

This week, identify your biggest stressors and take a look at how you are dealing with them. Do the stressors you've identified negatively affect your ability to make healthy food choices and be physically active? If so, use the space below to write down some ideas for healthier coping strategies that will not only reduce stress, but help you reach your weight loss goals and continue to practice self-care.

My Stressors	Current coping strategy	Healthier coping strategy
Job responsibilities	Happy hour after work	Walk with a colleague or friend
Commute to work	Eating fast food in the car	Eat Jenny Craig meal before driving and listen to Motivational Audio in the car.

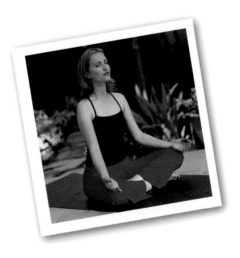

Weight Pessimist

Goal: Practice Optimism

Focus on the Positive

If you have made multiple attempts to manage your weight, you may have become a bit of a weight pessimist. If so, you might explain your history of weight gain, loss and re-gain in terms of what health experts call the "3 P's" – personal, pervasive and permanent. It's personal because you tend to blame your own lack of willpower, weakness or other character defect for your results. It could also be pervasive, because you've begun to transfer your feelings about weight to other areas of your life; you begin to think you lack willpower in all your endeavors, not just weight. And, it could be permanent, because it sometimes feels like the situation will never change – you'll always be battling your weight. What about the times when you do feel successful? If your "weight worldview" is more negative, you're more likely to give credit to a stroke of luck, rather than a stroke of your own genius or perseverance.

Mastering Optimism

Take heart. Experts say that while your weight loss worldview is partially programmed by genetics, you can shift your perspective with a little practice – and support.

That's why it's so important to surround yourself with people who believe in you – your Jenny Craig Consultant, close friends, family – those who will affirm all your positive efforts while you are learning how to do it yourself. One technique to help you get started on the path to learned optimism is called "reframing in the positive." Take a step back and look at the event in a positive way. For instance, if you don't lose weight one week, instead of viewing it as a "sign" that the Program isn't working, try a new spin. Focus on what is working. Give yourself credit for the positive changes you're making in your eating and activity behaviors. Acknowledge that these changes aren't the result of luck, but your own planning and commitment. Weight loss or not, you'll see that, based on your own positive efforts, it was a great week!

Keeping Track

Starting this week, look for ways to catch yourself being successful. Count up the meals and snacks you ate and crossed off on your menu, as well as the number of times you followed through on your activity plan. Think of it – 4 meals/snacks per day, 7 days a week, plus at least one opportunity a day to be physically active – that represents 35 times per week to be successful. Tally your healthy choices up and note them as "wins" on your weekly menu. Week by week, you can use a focus on the positive to lift the old cloud of doubt and make room for the positive expectation that you will achieve a healthy weight for life.

Diet Extremist
Goal: Practice Moderation

Focus on Moderation

When it comes to losing weight, do you take an "all or nothing" approach? If you do, you might feel as if you always are "on" or "off" a diet or exercise plan. You may also believe you need to follow a strict set of "rules" that dictate what, how much, and when you can (or cannot) eat, as well as how much, how intense and how frequently you should exercise. While the promise of rapid results makes this stringent style of dieting seem worth the sacrifice, it's this rigidity that actually works against you. Studies show that if you get bored, stressed or the urge for forbidden foods, you are more likely to react in a rebound "binge" that's as extreme as the diet.

Mastering Moderation

Experts say a better way is the middle way, a moderate approach that includes reasonable goals and flexes to your lifestyle and preferences. It starts with choosing a desired weight that is realistic for you and moves on to setting smart weekly goals that are specific, measurable and motivating. It also includes a menu that features your favorite foods, in moderate portions, as well as a plan for activity that builds on your current fitness level. This approach sets you up for progress, not perfection, where lapses are not the end of the world, but opportunities to learn how to create a more positive outcome.

Keeping Track

This week, be mindful of making moderate food and activity choices. When you plan a particular a Jenny Craig entrée or snack into your Menu, reassure yourself that, yes, you can enjoy your favorite foods and still lose weight. As you plan your weekly activity, know that it doesn't take a marathon, but several bouts, in a combination of natural, playful and planned ways, to burn calories and build your fitness level. Let the experience of taking small, planned steps toward a healthier lifestyle show you the value of a moderate approach to weight management.

Lifestyle Moderate

Goal: Maintain a balanced approach to living

Focus on Balance

Wonderful! Overall, you approach your weight with a very balanced mindset. You take a more self-accepting approach to your efforts, give yourself credit for your accomplishments and forgive yourself for your setbacks.

You have hopes for reaching your desired weight, and you are looking to make small, realistic changes, rather than drastic ones, to achieve your goals.

Mastering Balance

As you progress through your weight loss journey, we will continue to reinforce your balanced approach to living by offering you a variety of self-care and stress management strategies. You will also have the opportunity to focus on other areas of weight management related to Food and Body – such as learning how to eat for both health and weight loss and be physically active for life.

Keeping Track

This week, use your Menu as a convenient tool to self-monitor your progress and enhance your motivation. Not only can you compare your actual food intake and your physical activity to your weekly Plan, but you can also write in a Reward of the Month to as a way to stay inspired and support your self-care.

Support to Strengthen Your Healthy Weight Loss Mindset

Just as it takes practice to learn new eating and activity habits, it takes practice to develop a healthier weight loss mindset. As a start, experiment with the strategies offered in this Guide and the Weight Loss Manuals that follow, which are matched to the Weight Loss Mindset that was identified in the **Your**Style® Profile.

If you've long struggled with your weight, you might discover that you've been speaking to yourself in self-defeating ways for years. It may even seem unnatural to talk to yourself in any other way. That's why it's it helpful to have multiple resources for modeling healthy self-talk, ones that offer you positive thoughts over and over, to counteract the effect of the negative thoughts that have often been more familiar.

Often, it's just a subtle change in the language you use to talk to yourself about your weight that can motivate you to make a healthier choice. Know that you have the support of your Consultant, to reinforce the positive (and re-frame the negative) in your self-talk.

Along with the information in your program materials and the encouragement of your Jenny Craig Consultant, you have the support of two additional tools:

Jenny Craig's 28 to Motivate - a month's worth of quick strategies and affirmations that you can use to manage your unique weight loss challenges. Listen to one everyday – you'll be amazed at how energized and inspired you are to meet your goals.

This CD also includes a bonus "Help!" section, which give you quick tips to prevent a lapse or manage one so it doesn't become a relapse and you can stay on top of your goal.

Jenny Craig's Touchstones for Success™ – a motivational kit that uses a DVD, CD, and a set of touchstones that focus on five key strategies for transforming your weight loss mindset:

Becoming the Compassionate Witness

Learn how to let go of a self-critical, overly restrictive weight loss mindset.

Living From the Inside Out

Build your awareness of the power of internal versus external sources of motivation.

Putting First Things First

Learn how to make your weight a priority, even in the midst of conflicting demands.

Breaking the Binge Cycle

Learn how to use self-acceptance and self-care to manage and prevent lapses.

Enjoying the Moment

Re-discover the pleasure of food with this mindful eating experience.

By changing the way you think about weight loss, both **28 to Motivate** and **Touchstones for Success** can help you change what you do about it – steering your choices, your actions and your weight in the right direction.

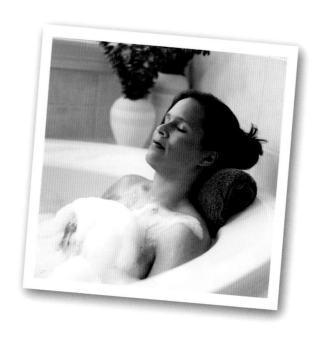

Mark Your Milestones

Revisit Your Motivation

One month into the program, how has your motivation to meet your goals changed? The short-term goal that inspired you the first few weeks of your program may be very different from the long-term goal that motivates you midway through your program. Now is a great time to re-visit your vision of why you want to lose the weight and refresh your motivation to succeed.

Celebrate Healthy Changes

Once a month, take time to reflect on all the ways there are to measure your success. Along with celebrating the pounds and inches lost, acknowledge the positive lifestyle changes you've made.

As you rate your confidence level for each food/body/mind behavior, use the number as a gauge to recognize your strengths and opportunities for building a healthy lifestyle.

Each Month…

- **Plot your weight** – celebrate both week and total pounds lost.
- **Take your measurements** – add up the inches that translate to a leaner, more toned body
- **Food:** Rate your confidence with healthy eating – are you ready to plan a meal on your own?
- **Body:** Rate your confidence with mastering your activity stage – based on your Personal Activity Quiz are you ready to advance to the next stage?
- **Mind:** Rate your confidence with stress management and self-care strategies – are you beginning to enjoy a more balanced lifestyle?

Reward Yourself

Lifestyle change requires effort that deserves to be honored. Rewarding yourself for your hard work can be very motivating. A reward is a (non-food) "treat" to yourself, above and beyond your usual self-care. Treat yourself to a manicure, bubble bath, massage, book or new CD. Use the "Reward" section on your menu to record how you will treat yourself as you reach your goals.

Ongoing Consultations

Stay Tuned In to Your Motivation

Each week, your consultant will ask you about the benefits you envision from losing weight and making positive changes. What motivates you? Is it:

- Looking good for an upcoming event?
- Fitting into a favorite outfit?
- Improving a health factor like cholesterol or blood pressure?
- Having the energy to take on more in your day?
- Enjoying the sense of pride you get from living healthfully?

Whatever that personal motivator is for you, keep it top of mind and influencing your positive choices, by writing it on your Menu and reading it to yourself every day.

Plan to Succeed With Your Menu

Successful weight loss doesn't happen overnight. It takes practice – and planning. People who successfully lose weight plan what they'll eat and how they'll be active on a regular basis. You can use your Menu to make a weekly plan that works for you.

Create a Realistic Plan

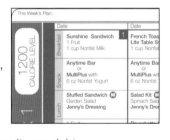

When you begin a weight loss program, you're motivated and excited to see results. That said, resist the temptation to set goals that may be unrealistically high. After all, it took months, maybe even years, to arrive in centre at your current weight. Just as you didn't gain your weight overnight, it's not realistic to expect to lose it overnight.

To ensure your success, talk through your weekly plan with your consultant, and set a goal that is specific, realistic, motivating – and measurable.

There are a variety of skills, strategies and information that can help you achieve your weight loss goal. Whether it's an aspect of Food, Body or Mind, your consultant will ask you to share your priorities and identify "This Week's Plan," so that you can get the most from your Program. Your plan can be something you do, like practicing a new dining out strategy or increasing the number of steps you walk or it can be beginning to think differently, like changing from negative to positive self-talk.

Focus on the Benefits

In deciding on a Plan, remember to think about why it's important to you. Beyond an action that will take you closer to your ultimate weight goals, think of the other benefits (health, appearance, relationships, etc). as well as the feelings (energy, confidence, sense of control, etc). that completing your Plan will bring. Both your benefits and feelings can motivate you throughout the week — providing you stay in touch with them.

To do that:
• Note your personal motivator in the **My Motivation** section of the Menu
• Read it often, visualize the benefits and imagine the feelings that remind you to make healthier choices throughout your day.

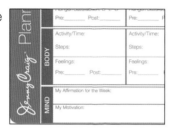

Know Your Challenges

Even the best intentions have potential obstacles. When you think about your plan, take a moment to honestly assess who or what could get in your way. What is it about the plan that is most difficult for you? It may be skills, strategies or even communication skills that could solve your challenge. Share your concerns with your Consultant so that you can set yourself up for a successful outcome.

Rate Your Confidence

Once you create a plan, your consultant will ask you to rate, on a scale from one to five, how confident you are that you can follow through with it. Don't worry. It's not a test, but a powerful tool to build your healthy lifestyle skills. If you rate yourself three or higher, it's a great indicator that you have built a realistic plan or that you are getting more competent in weight management every week. What if you rate your confidence less than a three? Maybe you'll want to re-evaluate your plan, perhaps it's overly ambitious. Or, if the plan seems realistic but you're having self-doubts, talk it over with your consultant. You may just need a little reassurance that you can do it.

Evaluate Your Plan

Each week, expect your Consultant to ask what parts of your plan worked – and what parts didn't. It's a great opportunity to recount successes and troubleshoot the challenges. Remember to bring your menu back to the consultation. If you've used it as the food/body/mind self-monitoring tool it can be, you'll have a ready-to-go recap of your week to share with your Consultant, which can help guide your plan for the upcoming week. Depending on your area of focus, you'll want to track one of these:

Food
- The Jenny Craig Menu foods you eat
- Extra Foods Eaten/Why
- Hunger and Satisfaction ratings

Body
- Activity/Time/Steps:
- Feelings Pre/Post

Mind
- My Wins for the Week

Affirm Yourself

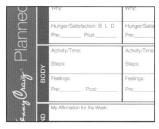

It takes time to change the way you believe and behave around weight issues. Along with a solid plan in which you have confidence, it's motivating to mentally reinforce it by practicing strong, positive self-talk. Affirmations are a vehicle to do that. They set you in a positive direction and help you see the best side of yourself. And the more good you find in yourself, the more you trade self-judgment for self-acceptance, the more open you are to taking risks and making changes.

Affirmations are most powerful when they are personal. You can either create your own affirmation or use one from your *28 to Motivate* audio or *Touchstones for Success* kit. Here are some examples:

My Affirmation
My goal is progress, not perfection.
I am responsible for my own success.
Compassion is my touchstone to freedom.
I turn lapses into learning opportunities.
Priorities are my touchstone to results.
Each healthy choice takes me closer to my goal.

Jenny's Grocery List

Use this guide to incorporate your favorite foods into your menu!

Vegetables

Non-starchy vegetables are Free (see "FREE FOODS" list), so it's okay to eat extras, but be sure to get at least three servings per day. Starchy vegetables (corn, peas, potatoes, winter squash, yams) can be found under "Starches."

Raw vegetables/Garden Salad . . . . (1 cup)
Cooked vegetables . . . . (½ cup)
Vegetable juice . . . . (½ cup/4 oz)

Fruits

Approximately 60 calories and 15g carbohydrate per serving

Fresh fruit . . . . (1 small to medium piece,
. . . . 1 cup berries, grapes or cut fruit)
Grapefruit, mango, papaya . . . . (½)
Plums, tangerines . . . . (2)
Canned fruit . . . . (½ cup)
Dried fruit/raisins . . . . (¼ cup)
Fruit juice . . . . (½ cup/4 oz)

Meats and Meat Substitutes

Lean Meats = 1 Meat

Approximately 35-55 calories, 7g protein and <3g fat per serving

Beans and lentils . . . . (½ cup = 1 meat + 1 starch)
Beef, USDA Select or Choice grades trimmed of fat
   (round, sirloin, flank, tenderloin, chuck roast,
   T-bone, porterhouse) . . . . (1 oz)
Cheese, fat-free or lowfat . . . . . . (1 oz or ¼ cup shredded
. . . . or 1 ¼ inch cube)
Cottage cheese, fat-free or lowfat . . . . (¼ cup)
Egg whites . . . . (2)
Egg substitutes . . . . (¼ cup)
Fish . . . . (1 oz)
Hot dog, fat-free or lowfat . . . . (1 small hot dog/1 oz)
Jerky (turkey, pork or beef) . . . . (½ oz)
Lamb (roast, chop, leg) . . . . (1 oz)
Parmesan cheese . . . . (2 Tbls grated)
Pepperoni, lowfat/turkey . . . . (½ oz, 2-3 slices)
Pork (tenderloin, chop) . . . . (1 oz)
Poultry, skinless . . . . (1 oz)
Shellfish . . . . (1 oz)
Tofu, light . . . . (¼ cup)
Tuna . . . . (¼ cup)

Meats and Meat Substitutes (continued)

Higher Fat Meats = 1 Meat + 1 Fat
Approximately 75-100 calories, 7g protein and > 3g fat per serving

Beef (ground, corned beef, Prime grades
    such as Prime rib, filet mignon) . . . . (1 oz)
Cheese, regular . . . . (1 oz or ¼ cup shredded
. . . . or 1¼ inch cube)
Egg . . . . (1)
Fish, fried . . . . (1 oz)
Hot dog . . . . (1 small hot dog/1 oz)
Lamb (rib roast, ground) . . . . (1 oz)
Pepperoni. . . . . (½ oz, 2-3 slices)
Poultry, with skin or fried . . . . (1 oz)
Pork (top loin, cutlet, butt, spareribs, ground) . . . . . (1 oz)
Tofu . . . . (¼ cup)

Milks

Nonfat Milks = 1 Milk
Approximately 90-110 calories,12g carbohydrate, 8g protein and <3g fat per serving

Milk, fat-free or 1% . . . . (1 cup/8 oz)
Soy milk or buttermilk, fat-free or lowfat . . . . (1 cup/8 oz)
Yogurt, fat-free, light (sugar-free) . . . . . . (1 container/6 oz)

Higher Fat Milks = 1 Milk + 1 Fat
Approximately 120-150 calories, 12g carbohydrate, 8g protein and >3g fat per serving

Chocolate milk, 2% or whole . . . . (1 cup/8 oz)
Milk, 2% or whole . . . . (1 cup/8 oz)
Soy milk or buttermilk, full-fat . . . . (1 cup/8 oz)

Alcohol

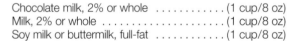

Approximately 90 calories per 2 Fat servings
Wine spritzer . . . . (5 oz, half wine/half soda) = 1 fat
Wine . . . . (5 oz) = 2 fat
Light beer . . . . (12 oz) = 2 fat
Distilled spirits . . . . (1 ½ oz) = 2 fat
Beer, regular . . . . (12 oz) = 1 starch, 2 fat
Martini . . . . (2 ½ oz) = 3 ½ fat

Fats

Approximately 45 calories and 5g fat per serving
Mono- and Polyunsaturated (choose more often)
Avocado . . . . (⅛)
Margarine, soft, regular . . . . (1 tsp)
    reduced-fat/light . . . . (1 Tbl)
Mayonnaise, regular . . . . (1 tsp)
    reduced-fat/light . . . . (1 Tbl)

Fats (continued)

Nuts . . . . (4 large or 10 small)
Oil (canola, corn, olive, peanut, safflower
    or soybean) . . . . (1 tsp)
Oil-based dressing, regular . . . . (1 Tbl)
    lowfat/light . . . . (2 Tbls)
Olives . . . . (8)
Peanut butter . . . . (2 tsps)
Seeds . . . . (1 Tbl)

Saturated (choose less often)

Butter, regular . . . . (1 tsp)
Cream cheese, regular . . . . (1 Tbl)
    reduced-fat/light . . . . (2 Tbls)
Creamy salad dressing, regular . . . . (1 Tbl)
    lowfat/light . . . . (2 Tbls)
Sour cream, regular . . . . (2 Tbls)
    reduced-fat/light . . . . (3 Tbls)

Starches

Lowfat Starches = 1 Starch
*Approximately 80-100 calories, 15g carbohydrate,
3g protein and <3g fat per serving*

Animal crackers. . . . . (8)
Beans and lentils . . . . (½ cup = 1 meat + 1 starch)
Bread . . . . (1 slice/1 oz)
Candy, hard . . . . (3 pieces)
Cereal, unsweetened . . . (¾ cup cold or ½ cup cooked)
Crackers, lowfat. . . . . (4)
Graham crackers. . . . . (3 squares)
Oyster crackers . . . . (24)
Pancake. . . . . (4-inch across x ½-inch thick)
Pasta sauce/marinara, lowfat. . . . . (½ cup)
Popcorn, lowfat/air-popped . . . . (3 cups)
Pudding, regular . . . . (¼ cup)
    sugar-free. . . . . (½ cup)
Rice or pasta. . . . . (½ cup)
Rice cakes . . . . (2, 4-inch across)
Roll, English muffin, pita, bagel
    or lowfat muffin . . . . (½ item or 1 oz)
Snack foods, lowfat . . . . (½-1 cup or ¾-1 oz)
Soup, tomato, split-pea, broth-based
    or lowfat cream-based . . . . (1 cup/8 oz)
Starchy vegetables (corn, peas, potatoes,
    yams and winter squash such as acorn,
      butternut, pumpkin and spaghetti) . . . . (½ cup)
Tortilla . . . . (6-inch)

Starches (continued)

Higher Fat Starches = 1 Starch + 1 Fat

Approximately 125-145 calories, 15g carbohydrate, 3g protein and >3g fat per serving

Biscuit . . . . (2 ½-inch across)
Brownie or cake, unfrosted . . . . (2-inch square)
Cookies . . . . (2 small)
Corn bread . . . . (2-inch square)
Crackers . . . . (4)
French fried potatoes . . . . (16-25/3 oz)
Granola bar . . . . (1.3 oz)
Hummus . . . . (⅓ cup)
Ice cream, light . . . . (½ cup)
Muffin or cupcake . . . . (½ item or 1.5 oz)
Pasta sauce/marinara, higher fat . . . . (½ cup)
Popcorn, microwave . . . . (3 cups)
Snack foods, regular . . . . (½-1 cup or ¾-1 oz)
Soup, cream-based . . . . (1 cup)
Stuffing, bread (prepared) . . . . (⅓ cup)
Waffle . . . . (4-inch square or across)

Combination Foods

Approximately 340 calories per 1 cup serving

Burrito (7-inch tortilla) . . . . 3 starch, 2 meat, 3 fat
Casserole, chili or pasta
   with meat sauce (1 cup) . . . . 2 starch, 2 meat, 2 fat
Energy, sport or breakfast bar (1 ⅓ oz) . . . . 2 starch, 2 fat
Pizza, thin crust (2 slices/ ¼ of 10-inch)
   meatless . . . . 2 starch, 2 meat, 2 fat
   with meat topping . . . . 2 starch, 2 meat, 3 fat
Pie, fruit (⅙ of an 8-inch) . . . . 3 starch, 2 fat
   pumpkin or custard (⅛ of an 8-inch) . . . . 2 starch, 2 fat
Soy or vegetable burger (no bun) . . . . 1 starch, 1 meat
Sushi, California roll (6 pieces, 2" x ½") 2 starch, 1 meat, 2 fat
Taco (6 to 7-inch tortilla) . . . . 1 starch, 2 meat, 2 fat

FREE FOODS

Approximately 0-30 calories per serving
Unlimited

• **Free Beverages:** Coffee, Tea, Diet Soda, Diet Tonic, Club Soda, Carbonated or Mineral Water, Sugar-Free Drink Mixes(0 calories). If you choose to decrease your caffeine intake, do so *gradually*.

• **Sugar Substitutes:** Equal,® Splenda,® Sweet'N Low,® Sweet One® (0 calories)

• **Gelatin Dessert, Sugar-Free** (0-10 calories)

• **Gum, Sugar-Free** (0-10 calories)

• **Flavor Enhancers:** Bouillon/Broth (low-sodium), Catsup, Extracts, Garlic, Herbs (fresh or dried), Horseradish, Lemon Juice, Lime Juice, Mustard, Pickles, Pimiento, Salsa, Spices, Soy Sauce (light), Taco Sauce, Vinegar, Worcestershire Sauce (0-25 calories).

• **Non-Starchy Vegetables:** Artichoke, Asparagus, Beans (green, wax, Italian), Bean Sprouts, Beets, Broccoli, Brussels Sprouts, Cabbage, Carrots, Cauliflower, Celery, Cucumber, Eggplant, Greens (collard, kale, mustard, turnip), Jicama, Leeks, Mushrooms, Okra, Onions, Pea Pods, Peppers (all varieties), Radishes, Salad Greens (endive, escarole, lettuce, romaine, spinach), Sauerkraut, Summer Squash (crookneck, yellow), Tomatoes/tomato paste/tomato sauce, Turnips, Vegetable Juice (low-sodium), Water Chestnuts, Zucchini (10-25 calories).

Limited (May choose up to 3 servings/day)

• **Whipped Topping or Syrup, Sugar-Free,** 1 Tbl (10-25 calories)

• **Jenny's Cuisine™ Lite Table Syrup,** 1 packet (35 calories)

• **Candy, Sugar-Free,** 1 piece (10-20 calories)

• **Fat-Free Condiments,** 1 Tbl: Cocoa Powder, Cream Cheese, Jelly (low-sugar), Margarine, Mayonnaise, Non-Dairy Creamer, Salad Dressing, Sour Cream (10-30 calories)

• **Fruits,** 1/2 cup: Cantaloupe, Strawberries, Watermelon (20-30 calories)

Note: Your actual calorie level may vary based on your food selections and number of "free food" choices.

Visual Cues for Serving Sizes

1 tsp. . . . . quarter, tip of thumb

1 Tbl . . . . silver dollar, whole thumb

2 Tbls (⅛ cup) . . . . . . one sandwich cookie, nailpolish bottle

¼ cup (4 Tbls) . . . . golf ball, large egg

⅓ cup. . . . . compact, espresso cup

½ cup . . . . ½ orange, small fist

1 cup . . . . baseball, light bulb

1 oz meat/cheese . . . . computer disk, tube of lipstick

1 oz snack food. . . . . rounded handful

2 oz meat/cheese. . . . . 3 fingers, 4 dominoes

3 oz meat/cheese. . . . . deck of cards, computer mouse

4 oz meat/cheese . . . . palm of man's hand

1 muffin or piece of fruit . . . . tennis ball

1 bagel . . . . 6-oz can of tuna

Your Pathway to Success

At Jenny Craig, we know you are looking for the key essentials of weight management to set you up for long-term success. Your Food, Body, Mind and Milestone consultations are pivotal to your program.

Your Food Consultation:
Your consultant will partner with you to develop a balanced eating style and design a menu that reflects your personal lifestyle and personal tastes.

Your Body Consultation:
Your consultant will offer you new strategies to help you master your current physical activity stage and move on to the next to gradually build a more active lifestyle.

Your Mind Consultation:
Your consultant will support you in developing the healthy weight loss mindset that can motivate you to create the healthy lifestyle and meet your desired goals.

Your Milestone Consultation:
You and your consultant will take time to reflect on your wins over the past few weeks and celebrate all your healthy changes. Your consultant will also show you how to create weekly plans that work for you.